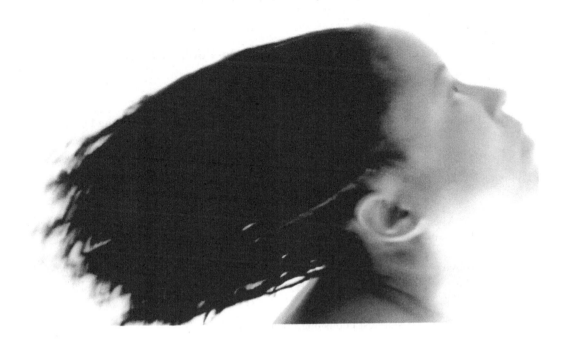

The Knotty Truth: Creating Beautiful Locks on a Dime!

A Comprehensive Guide to Creating Locks

The information contained in this book is based upon the research and personal and professional experiences of the author and reflects the author's professional opinion. The publisher does not advocate the use of any particular healthcare protocol or product but believes in presenting this information to the public. For further exploration of individual product lines, seek information from that manufacturer. This manual does not seek to endorse any product line. Should the reader have any questions concerning the appropriateness of any procedures or preparation mentioned herein, the reader should consult a professional healthcare advisor.

Library of Congress Cataloging-in-Publication Data

George, M Michele

The Knotty Truth: Creating Beautiful Locks on a Dime! A Comprehensive Guide to Creating Locks. M. Michele George.-1st ed.

p. cm.
Includes bibliographical references and index.

Published in the United States by Manifest Publishing Enterprises

1. African american women-Health and hygiene. 2. Hairdressing of African Americans. 3. Hairdressing of Blacks. 4. Hair-Care and hygiene. 5. Beauty, Personal. Dreadlocks. I. Title.

ISBN-13: 978-0-9832625-0-3
ISBN-0983262500

Printed in the United States of America

Editing Team:
Medical Editor: Deidre Redd, MD
Creative Editor: Brenda Robinson
Literary Critique and Editor: Aquila Butler
Policy and Ministerial Editor: Ronald George
Cosmetology Consulting Editor: Queen Roshae
Biomedical Assessment Editor: M Michele George

First Edition

Dedication

<u>Dedicated to my parents</u>
<u>Myron & Brenda</u>

<u>Dedicated to my guys</u>
<u>Ron, Josh and Jordan</u>

<u>Dedicated to my</u>
<u>Grandma Gin</u>
for all you poured into me
for the mantle you rested upon me
I hope you are proud.

CONTENTS

Creating Beautiful Locks on a Dime!

This book is great! I ordered for my daughters and read this book in one day. I could NOT put the book down. It is packed with helpful information related to how to lock natural hair. I wish I had this book when I first became a dad, it would have made hair washing day so much easier! The author has definitely gotten to the root of natural hair and this book will give an appreciation for our hair and how to handle it. I highly recommend the whole book series to all dads with daughters!
- *M. Rodney Robinson, Sales Manager Facebook*

A must-read for anyone contemplating holistic hair care free of chemicals. With The Knotty Truth series of natural hair care books, I am finally armed with information to care for our hair! As a medical professional, The Knotty Truth series is a refreshing alternative that I will share with my patients and friends! With this new addition on hair locking, I am armed with even more knowledge to care for my family's hair; but, also to direct patients who require alternatives that are healthy and good for their body.
-Dr. Dawn McCoy, MD

The Knotty Truth is one of those works that transports the reader from the writer's journey directly into her own. Women of all ages, in all stages of the natural journey and ones who have not yet begun their own will thoroughly enjoy reading this book. As I read, I was transported to different stages of my own life experiences as a loose natural and locked. I realized again that all of us have stories to tell and wisdom to impart. Having struggled with the concept of natural hair in America and internationally, while conversing with hundreds of women about their hair and identity struggles, I have found that creative and informational resources such as The Knotty Truth are like gold. Through these works, we realize we are not alone in our journeys our thoughts and feelings. I thoroughly enjoyed The Knotty Truth and I recommend it as a thoughtful, deeply moving and valuable read.
-Patricia Gaines aka Deecoily, Executive Founder, Nappturality

This sista gets it. It's about each one reach one. With each publication Sister Michele comes out hard and she comes out strong. Finally, setting the record straight on the care of nappy hair, The Knotty Truth has helped me during my consultations to educate those who need to know about the care of loose natural hair and now compliments my efforts with my lockers interested in different forms of locking. She plainly puts what the village has passed down on paper for the future to reference. Now, another generation can step the game to the next level. I thank you my sister. Ashe.
-Queen Roshae, Licensed Cosmetologist

Acknowledgements

This book is dedicated to all the naturals around the world that participated in this project. This project is possible because it is a collective effort from a family of naturals that believe in the village concept of each one teach one. Thank you for sharing that 'creating beautiful locks on a dime' is no secret. We are blessed to be a blessing. Thank you for heeding the call.

This book is dedicated to the men in my life. My husband, Ron, for always believing in me, cheering me on, working as my publicist, marketing team and promoter. My sons Josh and Jordan for encouraging me to finish this project. You understood when I had to cook with the lap top open, help you with your homework, while editing, wait for you at your practices while typing, I thank you for your patience with me. You shared me, encouraged me and cheered me on. It meant the world to me when a mother's guilt tugged at me; yet, you never let on that you minded.

To my mother and father for always showing me how proud you are of me. You shared with everyone that your daughter is an author, and showered me with your surprise of the acclaim of *The Knotty Truth* books! The respect, accolades and praise you showered upon me is appreciated. To my mother who supported me with articles, editing expertise and the greatest form of flattery: imitation by following me with your own lock journey, I thank you for your love, time and attention to creative detail.

To my awesome editing team, I trusted you with my baby and you gently handled her, nurtured her, cared for her and gave her back to me, better than when she left. Thank you for your time and commitment to this project. I thank the world-wide audience known and unknown that supports this project, bought The Knotty Book books, and attended the seminars and workshops. Thank you!

FOREWORD

CREATING BEAUTIFUL LOCKS ON A DIME!

This comprehensive guide to creating locks is not just about cultivating beautiful locks, economically. This book takes *The Knotty Truth* to another level by incorporating the art of holistic hair care with the art of locking highly textured hair. Holistic hair care is the art of using and implementing organic, natural ingredients that are healthy and whole for the body and hair. This manual integrates the care and the unique science of hair texture properties with the art of locking, creating a foundation to create beautiful locks with everyday kitchen ingredients that are edible and healthy.

This guide is necessary as the incident of cancer has increased in the general population, and the modernization of our society has brought on a daily, weekly, monthly and yearly accumulation of toxins from beauty and health care products; coupled with the onslaught of toxins in our foods and environment accumulating in our bodies, overloading our systems. This manual is necessary, because cosmetology licensing does not differentiate between holistic hair care products that are 'green' and healthy for the environment and our bodies[1] and commercial products laden with chemical toxins like formaldehyde, parabens and aluminum. Further, the study of 'nappy[2]' hair is not taught in beauty school simply because it is not on the licensing test. In the twenty-first century, the standardized cosmetology books, used by beauty schools, continue to teach that highly textured hair is coarse and unmanageable, needing to be relaxed, transforming highly textured hair to straight hair, the industry standard. All stylists and clients have the right to know how to care for highly textured hair, creating locks with the utmost care with this unique texture, in a tangible written format. This manual is an extension of this effort being the first of its kind, addressing this untapped niche, with detailed instructions, visual details, studies, personality, lifestyle and professional charting to help the locker decide the best way to create beautiful locks on a dime with conscious hair practices.

The industry standard that straight hair is ground zero must be redefined for highly textured hair. In actuality, ground zero for straight hair is a straight texture; ground zero for curly hair is a curly texture; ground zero for wavy hair is a wavy texture. Breaking down confusing barriers on the state, management and care of highly textured hair is vital as licensed professionals and the public seek to become more embracive of all people, of all hair textures, reigniting the hair care profession by equipping and empowering an untapped clientele. This second book in The Knotty Truth series: *Creating Beautiful Locks on a Dime!* will continue to empower the savvy customer to care and maintain his/her own locks in between visits or independent of visits.

This manual is my desire to change ground zero to a new standard that embraces highly textured hair by pushing the reset button. What we do with it from here is up to us. The knowledge is now spreading on YouTube, online forums like www.nappturality.com, blogs, books, tapes, workshops, seminars, DVDs, webinars, meetup groups, tweets, chats, texts, expos, certification programs, and there's no stopping it! These mediums are being used to circumvent an industry that has been less than embracive of 'nappy' hair by taking back control of what is considered 'unmanageable', 'coarse' and 'unworthy' via these unconventional, new-age mediums. More women are 'growing' chemically free hair for various reasons, becoming empowered. By working with the intricate design of highly textured hair, these conscious hair care books are written to consolidate and teach what is not taught in a traditional venue of learning. It's time that those who want the knowledge to seek and attain that knowledge without barriers. Those who choose to remain ignorant out of disdain or lethargy can attain from the established venues of traditional learning. The finish line now realigns the former with a new methodology that embraces the bend of highly textured hair with the following precepts:

- Nappy hair is manageable.
- Nappy hair is fragile, not coarse.
- All hair is not the same, and should be uniquely managed.

---

[1]Google these following toxins now or read in The Holistic Hair Care Chapter.

[2]The word nappy is synonymous with any reference to highly textured and curly hair in this manual. It is a positive word that embraces the tight kink of our hair and not meant to be derogatory in any way.

This manual is a compilation of many stories. Some of the written and pictorial stories are from individual lockers who have created beautiful locks at home. Other stories are shared by lockers whose locks are cared for by professional lockticians. Some of the stories are shared by actual licensed professionals who have gone the extra mile to learn the art of caring for highly textured hair beyond the auspices of cosmetology. Because they believe in this journey, they have been kind enough to contribute to this manual, as well. The pictures are a compilation of all contributors proving that locks can be created from the home to the salon. May you finally learn all you need to know about creating beautiful locks on a dime from start to finish for yourself!

*No information in this book may be reproduced without the author's written consent. When referencing materials, systems and theories, please give all credit to this author **M. Michele George, Certified Natural Hair Coach and Consultant**. The author actively travels presenting The Knotty Truth workshop as a CEU provider for licensed professionals as well as to the general public. If you would like a one on one training, in-service or workshop, please contact The By George! Team at cheleski@theknottytruth.net and www.theknottytruth.net for more information.*

PART ONE

THE FOUNDATION

Why Dread?

Why Lock?

The Reason!
The Introduction

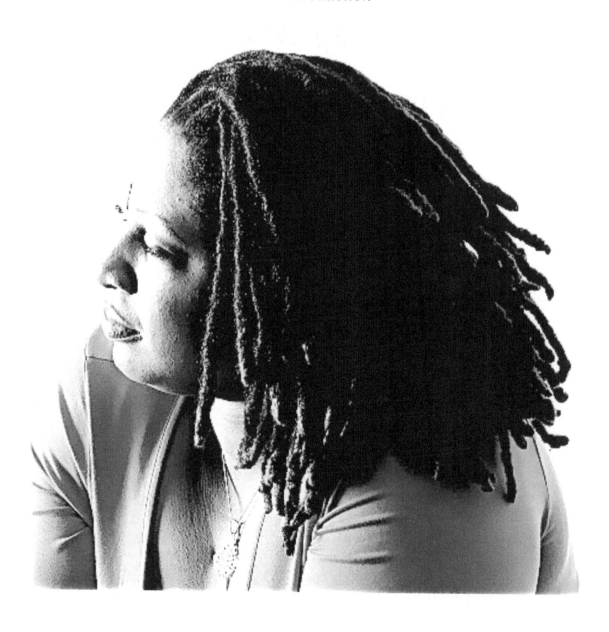

Once upon a time dreadlocks were not a popular hairstyle, relegated to only a few cultures like the Hermitic priests of Israel, the Himba of Namibia and Angola, some of the Hindu faith, tribes of Kenya, Islamic groups, Masai of Tanzania and other peoples of the globe as a form of cultural expression or spiritual growth. In the 20th century, dreadlocks became well known and affiliated with the Rastafarian of Jamaica. However, as the 20th century came to a close, dreadlocks have entered into the mainstream population as another form of self-expression. Dreadlocks can be seen in all shapes, forms and sizes from the micro-hair strand thin locks of Sisterlocks™ to the thick, organic free-form lock. There are locks in all shapes and forms with a la carte menus available from foundation to maintenance. Locking can be for deeply spiritual reasons or a personal style option. Because of these reasons, it's important for the locker to identify with a reason, because the why is the cornerstone that will anchor the locker into a solid foundation when the days get predictably stormy and rocky.

People lock for various reasons, for example: self-expression, fashion, a manifestation of ethnic pride, a political statement, spiritual reasons, a personal platform, or styling ease. Another benefit of locking is personal and emotional growth. Many lockers find that locking can take them on a surprising journey to self-awareness, because a spiritual awakening may occur. In the 21st century, it's not uncommon to find lockers who don't lock for spiritual reasons; however, many do hold to the historical, spiritual and sacrificial meaning of locks. Not all lockers are spiritual; however, acknowledging the spiritual foundation of dreadlocks is important, regardless of one's position, because the history of dreadlocks is born out of a story that reaches beyond the physical, becoming multidimensional. Just in case the locker encounters die hard lockers along a spiritual path, or the path diverts and takes a spiritual turn, it's important to understand the origins of this journey and the implications it can have on the locker's life and those involved.

The 'why' will help the locker get through the rough days that will come as the hair sprouts, buds, frizzes and mats by giving the process purpose and function. For many, locking is a journey. However, not all journeys may have roots in a spiritual evolution, for all it is unique. The locker must identify the why, the reason to lock. The why will carry the locker through the low points when friends and family fail to understand why "You won't take a comb to your head and straighten that mess out." The why will carry the locker when s/he (she or he) is on that all important job interview wondering if the locks will be acceptable for hire. The why is the purpose! And, the why is personal.

Lockers often face criticism, disapproval and misunderstanding from Christian faith-based groups, which can be judgmental and ignorant of the rich Judeo-Christian origin of locking. The dreadlock journey even emerges from the pages of time with captivating stories of the locker Samson's bravery, courage, shame, maturation, growth, defeat, and cleansing. Biblical stories such as Samson and Delilah give examples of the rich heritage of locks among the Nazarites of the Old Testament Bible:

Judges 16

Samson, single handedly fought armies of Philistines and won! But, he had one weakness, women! Her name was Delilah and the Philistines bribed her into finding the source of Samson's power. His source was God and his source was his sacrifice,
"No razor should touch his head"
Samson had 7 locks that grew from his head, a number that signifies spirituality. Samson was a Nazarite from the Hebrew people, whose lives are dedicated, consecrated and separated to the Lord.

Samson's lock journey was grounded in a spiritual foundation of sacrifice and love for the Lord. From the Old Testament to the New Testament, references to matted hair can be found throughout the Bible, streaming through many faiths.

Locks have been a part of the history of almost every spiritual system from Christianity to Hinduism, becoming a symbol of a highly spiritual person who is trying to come closer to God. Priests of certain deities are known to sacrifice the combing of their hair for years, devoting their life to that deity. Tutankahamen and other Pharoahs locked their hair. These locks can still be found intact on the mummified hair of corpses. The Kemetic people, the oldest and most authentic spiritual order, believe in the seventy-seven commandments from The Great Book of Divine Ordinances: The Code of Human Behavior translated by Master Naba Lamoussa, and practiced today. The seventy-seven commandments are spiritual laws given to humanity from their Gods. Similar to Christianity, these 77 laws mirror the 10 commandments of the Bible and speak of treating others the way we would like to be treated.

Another well known example of how locks relate to a deep spiritual journey is the Rastafarian which means one who fears the Lord. The Rastafarian bible, the Pentateuch (the first five books of the Christian bible) express that locking is a form of sanctification and spiritual sacrifice from the Rastafarian to the Lord. Dreadlocks were also worn in Jamaica as a form of liberation from the dominant culture, England. Growing dreadlocks was born out of defiance and an intense desire to love self. Under British rule, a band of Jamaicans emerged full of grace and defiance against their oppressor after hiding in the forest hills for months preparing to take back their Island. In the middle of the 19th century, the exact period that the American Revolution occurred, Jamaica's oppressed Negro population began to rebel until 1962 when independence was granted. When the warriors emerged from the forests of Jamaica to defeat the oppressor, their locks were long and fashioned like that of a lion's mane. Word of fear and "dread" spread throughout the land. Rastafarians sacrificed their appearance by not combing their hair as their connection to Jah/ God intensified. The Rastafarian's spiritual revolution, turned personal evolution, turned political statement, come together, today, to express their monolithic identity.

As the art of locking has expanded from Africa to Asia, onward to Europe and the West Indies through people of Israel, India and the Middle East, to the Americas, locks have sprouted from the tops of heads adorning the crown of all hues, cultures and peoples for many reasons, usually as a form of self-expression which renounces the status quo, carving out uniqueness that characterizes individuality and distinction. Many lockers have shared that they feel more attune with their thoughts and the thoughts of others. Some feel closer to the creator, with an overwhelming proclivity to tap into their own inner peace and higher spirituality than before locking. As a result, the need for outward affirmations and compliments are minimized. Spiritual confirmation often intensifies, as physical self is minimized. Once the locker begins to leave the hair alone, time is freed up and a spiritual awakening may occur, as a restful state of being intensifies. The art of locking can be spiritual, beautiful, memorable and empowering, if the traveler is open to the journey and willing to be enlightened.

The physical process of locking from infancy to maturity is emotional, as well. The journey is not for the faint of heart, or those seeking a quick hairstyle. However, a beautiful thing about highly textured hair is that it will lock eventually. Extreme patience and endurance is required leading the locker towards exercising new gifts of awareness. While the physical journey of locking is occurring, there is a mental transition that quietly evolves. Those that choose to transition from a chemical process straight to locks can miss this part of the journey, because it is a multi-step process and can only be fully realized from taking the journey with unadulterated, chemical free hair. *The Knotty Truth: Managing Tightly Coiled Hair at Home* further explores how to mentally transition from chemically processed hair to natural hair with success, explaining three simple steps to break through the mental barriers of personal acceptance:

- See the vision
- Write down the vision
- Embrace the vision

The Knotty Truth: Creating Beautiful Locks on a Dime! delves into the mental and physical transition of accepting the beauty of locks at all stages while caring for them. To help along the mental journey, there is one key element essential to both the journey from chemical to natural hair, and from loose hair to locked hair: the village concept. Most travelers will need the village of sisters and brothers to affirm, share and grow with, whether that is the sharing of pictures, words of encouragement or an embrace that affirms to the new locker that each stage will soon pass. It's vital not to miss the lesson that comes with each pothole, detour and stop sign for true maturity to develop.

Sometimes locks are chosen as a hairstyle just for the physical ease of having them. Locks are known to be an excellent protective hairstyle that is low maintenance, with minimal manipulation. Many Lockers will express that they don't "get" all the hype of locking being a spiritual journey, evolution, or political statement. Some just want a change in hairstyle. That's fine! Life is a journey, for some hair is not. Those that choose to lock for the simplicity of the hairstyle may feel that hair will grow and hair will go! For many, like myself, locks evolved into a journey that has become both spiritual and personal. The advantage of this low maintenance hairstyle is the beauty of its simplicity. Locks are cords of matted hair that are not combed. If the hair texture is inherently tightly coiled, a comb can be a weapon to the hair. A deadly weapon that can cause damage or even death, as it has the ability to split the delicate cuticle, breaking open the hair strand to the core if improperly used! To prevent this damage, locks can be worn as a permanent protective hairstyle. The advantage of locks is that the hair does not need to be detangled. The hair can be washed, styled and braided without a comb, because the hair always stays in its matted, protective chord!

To deal with the emotional journey of growing a healthy head of locks and the physical testing of the journey, it's essential to come to terms with the terminology associated with locks. There has been controversy surrounding the word dreadlock because of the negative connotations that have been associated with dreadlocks post African Slave Trading. In the beginning of the 14th century with Portugal and ending in the 18th century with America, captured Africans emerged from the hulls of slave vessels into a new land. The European natives criticized the "dreadful" hair that was matted and embedded with filth and insects from months spent in crowded quarters. Excrement, sweat, blood and stomach bile formed an encrusted encasement that was integrated within the matted hair. The trauma of the Middle passage was manifested through the hair's "dreaded locks." This imagery stuck with Europeans and Africans alike. For the first time, the African regarded his/her hair as a crown of shame, and shadow of its former glory and for the first time in history, the African began to see their hair as something different and bad. Abruptly taken from their country, the rituals, styling aids, specialized combs and customs, were lost to a strange new world that knew nothing of the "dreadful" hair. Generations continue today to embrace the shame that America's chains have thrust into the minds, spirits and souls of those born with a kink in the hair and a constant battle to accept it.

On the contrary, time and time again, those who adorned their heads with locks have been able to turn this albatross of shame into a crown of glory, embracing the power of the kink. Some reconcile that the word dreadlocks connotes all things bad, as it is an inherent testament of all things wrong with highly textured hair. However, others have embraced the negative connotations of this word. By embracing the word "dreadlocks" the locker is now allowed to turn the negative implications, of what is seen as bad, into a positive as s/he learns to love the locks for their history and power. In this manual, the word may be used interchangeably between, dreadlocks, locks, dreads, but the meaning and power is all the same. In this manual, locks are used interchangeably with the word dreadlock, with all respect and attributes, simply meaning matted hair! The politics of the language will be the locker's decision; choosing what s/he best identifies with is a personal decision.

The art of locking is more about heritage than dogmatic rules and methods. It is a history passed down through oral and visual interpretation from generation to generation, never before captured in a step by step 'how to manual.' Prior to this printing, the study of locks had been summarized and shared; but, never intricately explained, because it is an art form based largely on intuition and verbal directives. Locking is about listening to the hair and hearing the needs of the hair, then partnering this with the biological state of the hair and lifestyle choice. For every method, there are counter methods. For every method, there is an alternative choice predicated on personality and preference. Since we must start somewhere, let this be the foundation to build upon so that future generations can understand its basis, importance, and most importantly, how to create beautiful locks. There may be more than one way to do any given technique. Use this guide as a directive to build a foundation upon.

This journey has many ups and downs that are necessary for a head of healthy locks to form. The mental transition of seeing the beauty of the evolution, pushing the envelope of accepted and established visages of beauty, will occur in the midst of the lock journey. This will not only challenge those witnessing the evolution, but the locker's value system will be challenged to accept a new medium of beautiful. The locking process is fascinating and it can be beautiful to witness what the dead material of hair will do when left alone. When allowed to thrive and grow, unadulterated, locks take on a life form of their own with a personality that can direct the locker into submission as a new standard of beauty is established. Locking is for the strong willed person. Find the 'why' and the purpose will be close at hand.

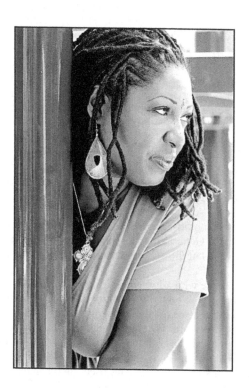

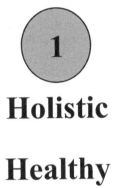

Holistic

Healthy

Hair Care

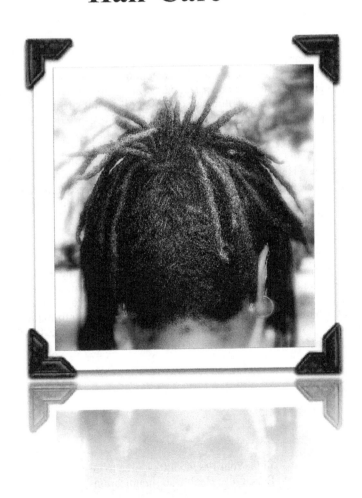

Edible hair care is healthy hair care that feeds the hundreds of hungry mouths inside of the scalp, affectionately known as hair follicles. Edible hair care is good for the hair and the budget, usually made with ingredients that serve a dual purpose of being edible for the scalp and the body. There are more than 100,000 chemicals in use in different areas of life and less than 5 percent of these chemicals have been thoroughly tested for their long-term impact on human health[3]. It's important to be aware of what is being put in the body, literally and figuratively. Toxic pollutants, nitrogen, carbon dioxide, oxygen and everything put on the skin's surface enter sweat ducts, hair follicles and sebaceous glands, directly entering the blood system, impacting the body.

Unfortunately, the health and beauty industry is not regulated to ensure the safety of a product before it is used on the market. For now, the industry monitors itself, making the politics of health and beauty skeptical at best. The public is the test market and personal care products are deemed safe until proven otherwise, according to the FDA. The US Food and Drug Administration (FDA) will only investigate health complaints after an accumulation of complaints have been filed. If the complaint reaches the investigation level, actual human data is hard to obtain from manufacturers. Becoming educated on what to stay away from is extremely important because the scalp has the richest blood supply in the entire human body. Whether locked, natural, or chemically relaxed, we all need to be aware and concerned about what components flow right into the bloodstream, via the scalp, to target organs in the lymph tissue and organs.

Because different products work differently for different people, it's important to understand why certain hair products and specific ingredients react differently on the hair. The effectiveness of hair products is impacted by the hair's genetic instructions, the DNA, which dictates the characteristics of hair: the density, texture, color, growth cycle, and length as well as seasonal and climate changes. Density of the scalp determines if the hair is thick or thin, because thick or thin hair will react differently to different amounts and types of products. Thick hair reacts well to butters, heavy emollients and oils like shea butter and castor oil. Thin hair reacts well to light oils like jojoba. It does not mean that heavy oils cannot be used on thin hair or a light oil on thick hair; however, the amount of product used and the way it spreads or pools on the hair may need to be adjusted because of these unique differences.

Porosity is an important indicator of the hair, because the more moisture a hair strand can hold, increases the hair's ability to expand and contract. Highly textured hair is already very porous, adding a humectant will further make the hair swell, expand and cuticles lift, remaining open and dry[4]. However, countering humectants with a sealant can seal in the benefits, thus sealing and protecting moisture levels. Use this combination to reap the benefits of moisture, manageability and luster.

Finding the right ingredients for the hair is important for highly textured hair, because it requires external and internal hydration and nourishment. Sebum is naturally produced in the scalp and provides nourishment and protection to the hair by forming a waterproof barrier for the hair and skin. The wax esters, triglycerides, fatty acids and squalene in the sebum, prevent the hair and skin from cracking and drying out, because they are natural emollients. However, it is hard for the sebum to travel down the tight curly formation of the hair. The oil cannot flow freely down the hair strand, as with straight hair. If oil is not added to highly textured hair, it becomes dry, looks dry, leading to damage as the hair strand's cuticle is compromised.

---

[3]Gabriel, Julie. The Green Beauty Guide: Your Essential Resource to Organic and Natural Skin Care, Hair Care, Makeup, and Fragrances. Deerfield Beach, FL: Health Communications, 2008. Print.

[4]The State of The Hair Chapter

Highly textured hair should be massaged nightly with oil to replenish the oil supply to the hair to distribute the sebum down the length of the hair strand[5].

The pH of ingredients can also impact the hair. The pH is the power of Hydrogen potential of a product and ranges from 0 (acidic) to 14 (basic). An acidic (acid) pH range is 0-3.0, an alkaline (basic) pH range is 8.0-14.0, neutral products are at a pH of 7.0 in the middle.

14	Liquid Drano	Alkaline (soft, porous, melting hair, open cuticles)
13	Bleach	Alkaline
12	Soap	Alkaline
11	Ammonia	Alkaline
10	Milk /Magnesia	Alkaline
9	Tooth paste	Alkaline
8	Baking Soda	Alkaline
7	Water	Neutral
6	Hair*	Acidic
5	Hair*	Acidic
4	Hair*	Acidic
3	Soda	Acidic
2	Lemon Juice, Vinegar	Acidic
1	Battery Acid	Acidic (shiny, closed cuticles, hard, breakage)

Fig. 2.1
pH Scale of everyday products

Hair is strongest at a pH of 4.5-5.5. At this pH, hair is compact and is a normal size. Hair in the alkaline range (8-14) will swell, cuticles will open and the hair will become porous and dry. Swelling changes the shape of the hair, making it more susceptible to other forms of distress, such as dryness and cuticle damage. Chemical Relaxers and

[5]It's best to avoid moisture with baby locks, to prevent unraveling. Mature locks can be moisturized as needed.

JUST SAY NO LIST!

Ingredient	Product	Natural Replacement	Purpose	Biological Impact
sodium laureth/lauryl sulfates; ammonium laureth sulfate	shampoo/foaming cleansers	natural soaps	surfactant, bubbles	triggers cancer, proven to damage eye tissue (Scaife,1985; Neppelberg,2007)
DEA/MEA aka cocamide diethanolamine	shampoo/foaming cleansers	natural soaps	surfactant, bubbles	triggers cancer:1,4 Dioxane present (Niculescu et al. 2007)
petroleum (petrochemical)	pomades, conditioner,hair grease products	vegetable glycerine hair butters	condition, shine or gloss, thickener	suffocates hair, environmental toxin.
mineral oil (petrochemical)	moisturizer products/ conditioners	vegetable oils	condition, shine or gloss, thickener	suffocates, prevents Oxygen exchange
synthetic silicone (petrochemical)	gloss and shine	organic castor oil, plant based silicones	shine and gloss	suffocates, prevents Oxygen exchange
aluminum	hair die	henna	dye hair	linked to Alzheimers, poison, breast cancer, (Exley et al. 2007)
parabens:methyl paraben, propylparaben, butylparaben, benzoic acids, isobutyl p-hydroxybenzoatep-methoxycarbonylphenol	many products	essential oils	preservative, extend shelf life of product	Proven to cause cancer in mice. Found in breast tumor tissue (Darbre 2006, 2002).
synthetic fragrances, phtalates,dyes	shampoo,conditioners, moisturizers	essential oils for fragrance	smell and appearance	triggers asthma (Curtis 2004) reproductive cancer in children (Stahlhut et al. 2007)
propylene glycol/ethylene glycol/diethylene glycol /PEG	popular humectants	Aloe Vera gel	moisture, conditioner, thickener	toxic, contact dermatitis, linked to birth defects and reduced sperm count(Anderson et al. 1987)
imidazolinyl urea, diazolidinyl urea, phenoxyethanol formaldehyde, quarternarium-15	many products	essential oils, potassium sorbate, vitamin C, vitamin E, fenilight, feniol, suprapein, lemon peel oil, grapefruit seed extract	preservative, extend shelf life of product	triggers cancer

baking soda are alkaline, contributing to open cuticles, swollen hair strands and dryness with a pH range of 8-14. A product with an acidic pH of 0-6.0, such as lemon juice, will contract and close the cuticles. Closed cuticles appear shiny but are not optimal for hair health either. Water is basic and normally in the 7.0 pH range. Focus on products within an acidic pH range of 4-6 which is optimal. Balance and adjust with purified water or Aloe Vera juice before using. By using pH strips (local health food store, drug store), adjust accordingly to make the product more basic or acidic with an optimal reading of pH 4-6, adjust with ingredient of choice. When considering what products to use, there are plenty of ingredients to avoid for optimum hair and body health. Lock cultivation thrives with ingredients that are positioned to nourish the hair and heal the body. Unfortunately, many of the over the counter products have ingredients that are harmful. In *The Knotty Truth Part One*, the *Do Not Use* list was shared. That was the 2007 compilation. Since then, science continues to reveal even more potent ingredients that can be avoided for healthy hair and body care. The 2011 *Just Say No!* list is a compilation of the most common offenders in hair products used for all types of hair as of this printing.

Shampoo

When caring for the locks, it is important to use clean products free of residue. Residue inhibits locks from forming, and contribute to build up, be sure to concentrate on a residue-free shampoo. Hair should be washed every week, or as needed. It is a myth that locks should not be washed for weeks and months at a time. A clean scalp with clean hair is a must! Follow the careful instructions on how to wash for success in *The Shampoo Chapter*. If under the care of a stylist, please follow his/her instructions.

It's best to use products free of the sulfates: sodium lauryl sulfate (sls), sodium laureth sulfate (sles), because they can be drying to the hair and harmful to the environment. They are linked to blindness (Neppelburg, 2007) and leave residue on the hair which can further affect the hair cuticle. While referring to the *Just Say No!* list, look for shampoos that are traditionally made by a cold-process, an unrefined process made with saponified vegetable and organic essential oils. Saponification is the process of making soap. Soap that is beneficial to skin and hair has glycerine in it, unlike commercial soaps on the market which extract the glycerine during production. Soap without glycerin is drying and irritating to the skin and drying to the hair, not residue free, creating irritating dandruff by leaving perfume and residue behind.

Traditional real African Black Soap or natural soaps are perfect for cleansing locks. Real African Black Soap is not black. It is brown, crumbly and made of shea butter, cocoa pods, burnt banana leaves, palm oil, natural glycerin and excellent for moisturizing and cleansing the hair and skin naturally. Look for soaps in import stores, health food stores or online from vendors such as BoBeam at http://www.etsy.com/shop/Laquita33 who creates wonderful natural soaps with natural ingredients. Free of oils and full of nourishment, BoBeam's soap bar: Locs Scalp Stimulator is a nice option for infant/baby locks. Infused with moisture and follicle stimulators, BoBeam's soap bar: Lemon Drop is for teenage and mature locks that have matted and settled. These products clean and moisturize because they lack additives, fillers and softeners without hindering the locking process or irritating sensitive skin. Residue from fillers is bad for dreaded hair because of the matting process. If build up occurs on the inside of the lock from residue, it could lead to

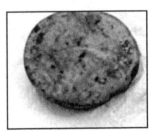

Real African Black Soap

mildew and fungus problems down the road, as it will form a breeding ground for germs to proliferate inside the matrix of the lock. Unfortunately, cloudy conditioning products have been linked to filmy, residual build up on locks. Test for residue by washing hands with the product. If it leaves a sticky, tacky feeling or a scent, residue is left behind. Another surfactant used to stabilize soap foams is the potentially carcinogenic diethanolamine (DEA) or methanolamine (MEA). These ingredients can synergistically combine with other chemicals in the body, leading to cancer (Niculescu et al. 2007). Avoid Shampoos high in moisturizers, proteins and chemical agents that give slip to the hair, which is good for detangling only, not for locks. If natural soap bars are not useful, look for commercial brands that will clean the hair, with little or no sulfates, while infusing moisture from nature with ingredients such as natural oils, essential oils and fragrances.

Becoming educated on the best ingredients to use and what to stay away from ensures optimal natural hair care. Whether using a commercial product line or natural products, this *Just Say No!* resource will be a guide for healthy hair and locks. Please use this as a resource. All liquid shampoo should be diluted in a spray bottle before using on locks. To a spray bottle, add a capful of shampoo to 8 oz of Aloe Vera juice or water, then spray into the hair and massage, then rinse for cleansing benefits. When looking for any product, natural preservatives are the best.

Humectants

Humectants are products that infuse moisture into the hair, nourishing the follicles and feeding the hair powerful nutrients. The purpose of a humectant is to add moisture to the hair. Humectants draw moisture to the hair during humid, warm months by allowing Oxygen exchange between the surface of the hair and the air. However, humectants detract moisture from the hair during the cool, dry months of fall and winter. Clear Aloe Vera (*Aloe barbadensis*) is a nourishing humectant in the pH range of 5.0-9.0. It has been used through centuries for wounds, irritations, skin infections and burns, rich in polysaccharides, galactose, plant steroids, enzymes, amino acids, minerals and even natural antibiotics. Adding humectants such as Aloe Vera gel, vegetable glycerine, jojoba oil, honey and lecithin fill in the pores of a hair shaft and feed the hair, while soothing and moisturizing the scalp. To keep the moisture in the hair, add a heavy emollient to close the cuticle to seal in the moisture[6]. For locks, humectants will feed dry locks moisture. The heavy oil/emollient will help to seal in that moisture. This combination coupled with a satin scarf will also reduce frizz and give some definition to hairline edges and styles that need a holding agent to set, adding shine. Other humectant options are glycerine, sorbitol, hyaluronic acid, honey among others.

Conditioning Mixtures

The most common offender for lock maintenance are products with mineral oil and petroleum, which is found in almost every lock-twist commercial gel preparation on the market. Not only is the product a barrier to Oxygen flow, it is hydrophobic. Hydrophobic products are not easily washed out of the hair, if at all. Hydrophobic means it repels water. Products with hydrophobic ingredients can lead to build up, discoloration and drying out of the hair. If used, the center core of the lock could appear white and flaky over time. The hair needs nourishing carrier oils to infuse nutrients into the cellular matrix of a hair cell. Hair cells are semi-permeable, which means they are part water 'loving' and water 'hating'. The nourishment is carried into a cell via a carrier oil which is comprised of lipids, fatty acids and other molecules. Focus on clear, natural, simple, hydrophilic products that help to bind loose strands together; such as the organic Aloe Vera gel/ conditioning oil mixture mentioned later in this chapter.

There is plenty of misinformation on the internet regarding the use of glue, and peanut butter, to bind locks. Avoid these products at all costs! Products that can help tame the frizzies without build up are simple, pure, natural and hydrophilic, water loving, such as a jojoba with a nourishing Aloe Vera gel combination. Aloe Vera gel is hydrophilic (dissolves easily in water) and will nourish, just fine. Substances such as shea butter and coconut oil are partially hydrophobic and hydrophilic and more difficult to wash from the hair, which may result in buildup, if not used properly; however, a better alternative than mineral oil or petroleum. Replace these ingredients with the nourishing conditioning and holding gel based in Aloe Vera gel, with honey (humectant) and an essential oil of preference (antioxidant, preservative). Aloe Vera gel nourishes the hair by feeding the hair precious healing nutrients that seep into the follicles. Aloe Vera gel also feeds the inner matrix, the core of the lock. As the lock is forming, Aloe Vera gel is absolutely critical to the health of the forming lock, preventing brittle, dry, dull locks by feeding hair from the inside out. Because Aloe Vera gel feeds the growing hair, beginning with a foundation bathed in Aloe Vera gel is not only healthy but cost effective, simple and easy! It's important to choose an Aloe Vera gel that is pure and organic. The best Aloe Vera gel must be refrigerated and never colored! No preservatives! If there are preservatives, opt for ascorbic acid, sodium benzoate or potassium sorbate as alternatives. Honey is proven to fight bacteria and fungi (Kwakman et al. 2008) and is a powerful humectant. Because honey is a strong allergen that should be used in its purest form to avoid any untimely chemical reactions. Commercial humectants such as propylene glycol and polyethylene glycol (PEG) are not toxic themselves; but, like sls and sles, they are laden with heavy concentrations of 1,4 Dioxane, polycyclic aromatic compounds, and heavy metals such as lead, iron, cobalt, nickel, cadmium, and arsenic contaminants[7]. Essential Oils act as preservatives and nourishment, while preventing product degradation. Be wary of their appearance in many commercial products.

---

[6]Once again, this applies to mature locks.

[7]Gabriel, Julie. The Green Beauty Guide: Your Essential Resource to Organic and Natural Skin Care, Hair Care, Makeup, and Fragrances. Deerfield Beach, FL: Health Communications, 2008. Print.

Preservatives

The purpose of a preservative is to extend the shelf life of a product. The obvious benefit is for the manufacturer, not the consumer. Therefore, it's more than wise to be savvy about the ingredients on health and beauty products, especially preservatives. So many preservatives are toxic and proven to cause cancer. Preservatives are rapidly absorbed, metabolized and accumulate in the human body. They are harmful because of their estrogenic characteristics which have been proven to cause uterine growth in animals and the growth of breast cancer cells (Darbe et al. 2002). In 1984, parabens were found to be harmful but deemed safe at levels of up to 25 percent of the finished product. To date, there are no cumulative human studies that show the impact of parabens chronically, because a sizeable population has not been found willing to be tested on an ingredient proven to cause tumors in rats. Parabens can be hidden as: benzoic acid, isobutyl p-hydroxybenzoate, p-methoxycarbonylphenol, methylparaben, propylparaben, butylparaben that all convert to parabens in the body. They are proven to cause cancer in mice and have been found in human breast tumors. Urea preservatives are a concern as well, listed as imidazolinyl urea and diazolidinyl urea. Ureas break down and form formaldehyde, the fixative for corpses that is proven to be carcinogenic. Phenoxyethanol is another preservative to avoid, because it breaks down into a formaldehyde, once inside the body.

There are healthy preservatives to look for, while shopping. As a preservative, essential oils prevent free-radical oxidation. Essential oils, without any contraindications for the locker, are always healthy alternatives; however, some can trigger negative responses like allergies, asthma. Seek products free of formaldehyde and ureas, sealed tight, in reduced light containers that inhibit bacteria, fungi, and yeast growth. Preparations made at home have a shorter shelf life, because of the natural preservative component, and lack of aseptic technique (sterile). Reduce contamination by keeping containers closed, tightly. Never use fingers, use an applicator stick, and discard within six months of opening. The following are a few examples of other healthy natural preservative alternatives:

Knotty Note

Natural Preservatives

fenilight
feniol
suprapein: thyme and oregano, cinnamon, lavender, lemon peel, goldenseal and rosemary extract
lemon peel oil
grapefruit seed extract
vitamin C (ascorbic acid)
vitamin E (tocopherols)
potassium sorbate
sodium benzoate

Knotty Note

Do not Use

petrochemicals: mineral oil, petroleum, silicones
sodium laureth/lauryl sulfates and other sulfate-based
detergents
propylene glycol, polyethylene glycol, PEGs and PGs
formulations
formaldehyde and paraben preservatives
synthetic (FD&C and other) dyes and colors
artificial fragrances

Synthetic Fragrances

Whether synthetic or natural, anything that is aesthetically pleasing (or not) to the nose may cause allergies. Most fragrances are never tested for safety and contain high levels of EtOH (ethanol, which is alcohol). Alcohol is drying to the hair. Fragrances are known to cause eczema, jawline dermatitis, acute contact dermatitis, and chronic actinic dermatitis (Wojnarowska, Calnan 1986). It's very important to pay attention to fragrances put in health and beauty products to enhance the smell. It's even better to avoid them altogether. There are too many health conditions that can result from exposure. Opt for fragrance free, or naturally flavored products. After learning and applying the new rules of engagement for holistic lock health care, it's time to complete the regimen.

Pre and Post Shampoo Rinse

Rinses serve different purposes. The pre and post shampoo rinse for locks is a rinse that will remove soap, scum, mineral deposits and product buildup from the locks, while sealing the cuticle, leaving the hair shiny. The Apple Cider Vinegar (ACV) rinse closes the cuticles because of its low, acidic pH! This will remove soap scum and help to neutralize the hair to its preferred pH range. The vinegar will also help to control dandruff and oily hair while adding shine, softness and bounce to the hair. Spray mixture into the hair, massage and let it sit for three to five minutes. Rinse out with warm water. Cleanse the hair, then rinse and follow up with conditioning solution.

Knotty Note

ACV Pre and Post Wash Rinse

Mix together in an 8 oz spritz bottle:

2 tablespoons lemon juice (15 drops) pH 2-3

1 pint of water pH 4-6 (will balance the vinegar and lemon)

¼ cup of Apple Cider Vinegar

Nourishing Herbal Conditioning Mix

Focus on clear, natural, simple, hydrophilic ingredients that will help to bind the loose strands together. Instead of conditioners with slip, opt for nourishing conditioning herbal teas like hibiscus, chamomile, green tea to feed the hair nourishing herbs full of rich nutrients that will feed the follicles and stimulate the roots. Chamomile is a herbal tea that lightens and nourishes the hair. Hibiscus Tea naturally colors grey hair with its dark, purplish dye. It soothes and cleanses the skin, rich in alpha hydroxy acids and amino acids, providing a tightening effect to the skin without stripping the natural oil. There are many nourishing benefits of herbal teas. Herbal Tea is perfect to condition new locks without ingredients that contribute to detangling. Herbal Teas infused into the nourishing conditioning gel, or use alone as a spritz will keep immature and mature locks nourished. Add half a cup of herbal tea to half a cup of Aloe Vera gel with 1 tablespoon of honey to the mixture for added moisture. Lemon juice can be added to further lighten the hair with 8 drops of preferred essential oil of preference. For follicular stimulation, a combination of rosemary and sage will synergistically aid in hair growth. Adding lemongrass will add a pleasing smell. Balance the pH with water to a range of 4.0-6.0 and apply to the head. Leave in and enjoy! Discard after use. The herbal tea can also be used alone as a leave in rinse or daily hair spritz, especially during the early months when locks are forming, to feed the hair.

Knotty Note

Nourishing Herbal Tea Conditioning Mix

1/2 cup Aloe Vera gel
1/2 cup preferred tea
8 drops preferred essential oil
1 tablespoon of honey

Nourishing Hair Spritz[8]

The purpose of a spritz is to nourish and feed the hair. Just as we feed our bodies via our mouth at meal time, it's appropriate to feed the follicle on the scalp as well, daily. This spritz is food for the hair. Spritzing can be done twice a day. Always follow up by massaging the solution into the scalp between applications. There are some Aloe Vera juices that can be stored room temperature, others must be refrigerated. For lockers with Type 1, 2, and 3 hair, mixing purified water with a pinch of sea salt, lemon juice or lime juice can make hair porous and prone to locking, if resistant (see Chapter two).

Healthy Hair Spritz

8 oz herbal tea
(1 tea bag, cup water)
8 drops of an essential oil
1 tsp jojoba
spray bottle
mix

Healthy Hair Spritz

8 oz Aloe Vera juice or purified water
8 drops of an essential oil
spray bottle
mix

Nourishing Hair Oil

The nourishing hair oil seals in moisture, by combining heavy emollients with lighter nourishing oils. Depending on the hair texture, density, mix an applicator bottle with one part castor oil and one part olive oil (or oil of preference). Some oils to use are nut oils like avocado, jojoba, lanolin, almond. Olive oil is a vegetable oil and all are known to feed the scalp and hair. Start simple with castor oil, a heavy oil, and organic extra virgin olive oil (OEVOO), unless there are allergies to ingredients in the oils. The nourishing hair oil will give definition, shine and moisture to thirsty locks. Remember the formula, Soften Feed Seal, as a solution for all moisture depraved, thirsty lock problems. S-soften/F-feed/S-seal will go a long way when locks become dry and unmanageable (Fig. 2.4)!

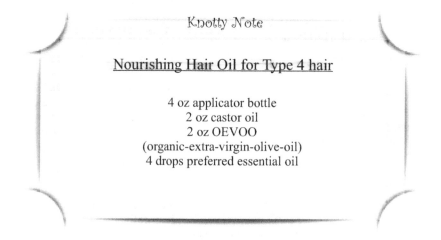

Knotty Note

Nourishing Hair Oil for Type 4 hair

4 oz applicator bottle
2 oz castor oil
2 oz OEVOO
(organic-extra-virgin-olive-oil)
4 drops preferred essential oil

---

[8]The best way to accelerate lock matting for baby locks is to make the spritz without oils and spritz frequently. After the locks have settled, feel free to add an oil component.

Vegetable butters are solid at room temperature, they are excellent sealers. Using butters such as kernel butters, coconut oil and cocoa butter can be tricky since they solidify at room temperature; furthermore, they may cause build up in locks if not properly used. Butters such as shea and cocoa butter should be used unrefined and cold pressed, because solvents are used in the refining process. Butters and oils are excellent carriers of nutrients across the cell membrane into the hair. The weight of an oil is determined by the specific gravity[9] of the oil; and, most have a healthy pH of 4-6. The higher the specific gravity, the heavier the oil. The heavier oils fair better on highly textured hair. The lighter oils fair better on straight and wavy hair. There are many carrier oils; however, the oils listed have excellent shelf lives and are moderately priced.

NATURAL OIL WEIGHTS		
LIGHT OIL	MEDIUM OIL	HEAVY OIL / EMOLLIENT
Jojoba	Sesame	Castor
Grapeseed	Sunflower	Coconut Oil
Almond	Palm	Glycerine
Advocado	Flaxseed	
Olive		
Emu		

Fig. 2.3 Carrier oils in accordance to specific gravity
*water has a specific gravity of 1.0

---

[9]Specific gravity is a measure of the weight of a liquid

HAIR TYPE	SOFTEN	FEED	SEAL
Type 1	Aloe Vera Juice	Light Oils	Light Oils
Type II	Aloe Vera Juice	Light Oils	Light Oils
Type III	Aloe Vera Juice	Light Oils	Medium Oils
Type IV	Aloe Vera Juice	Light Oils, Medium Oils	Heavy Oils/ Emollient

Fig. 2.4 Soften-Feed-Seal
Regimen
for four hair types

Stay focused on nourishing mature locks always. Baby to teenager locks can be more challenging to condition. The key with baby locks is to avoid the feed and seal method. Soften with aloe vera juice or conditioning herbal tea only! Rough, scratchy, dry locks can be touched up with jojoba oil from time to time if needed only.

BRINGING IT ALL TOGETHER
Commercial and DIY Options for Managing Hair

ACTION	SWEET NATURE BY EDDIE	FOXY LOCS	DIY*	ZURESH
PRE-RINSE			ACV rinse	
WASH	Natural Soap Bar	Clarifying Shampoo *for baby locks	Natural Soap Bar	
POST-RINSE			ACV rinse	
LEAVE-IN/ CONDITIONING		*Rinse out conditioner can be diluted. Conditioning moisturizer	Herbal Tea Conditioning Mix	Rebirth
ROOT TIGHTENING/HOLD	Follicle Stimulator mixed with Aloe Vera gel		Nourishing Conditioning and Holding Gel	Rebirth
FEED/SHINE	Follicle Stimulator		Nourishing Hair Oil	
SOFTEN/FEED	Growth Spray	Hair Oil	Nourishing Hair Spritz	Rebirth
SEAL			Castor Oil or Nourishing Hair Oil	

Fig. 2.5 http://foxylocs.com/index.html
http://www.fabulousblackwoman.com/index.html
http://www.zuresh.com/zuresh2/zuresh-main/main.asp?ssl=off
*DIY ingredients all purchased at local organic food store
disclaimer: This chart offers natural product lines with commercial
options available and used by the author. Experiences may vary.

The advantage of commercial products is the obvious ease of use. However, it's important to apply healthy hair care knowledge when using them. For example, if a product leaves a residue after washing, evaluate the efficacy for your hair, testing other options. If a creamy, conditioning product begins to leave build up, dilute it or switch to a self-maintenance alternative. Build up begins subtly. If a commercial product line, or a natural product line shows signs of build up, flaking, sticky residue, follow up with a deep cleansing treatment and a self-maintenance alternative.

There is no absolute best formula for every head of hair. There is only the best formula for one person's hair. Use Fig. 2.5 as the template, then add-on and tweak as needed for individual hair needs.

Healthy Food for Healthy Hair

Holistic lock health care would not be complete without incorporating healthy foods in the diet that attribute to strong roots and hydration from the inside to the outside of the body. Our skin and our hair manifest what is going on internally. Salmon, dark green veggies (spinach, broccoli, collards, kale), beans, eggs, nuts, oysters, yogurt and carrots provide excellent nutrients for strong hair. These foods contain zinc, iron, calcium, biotin, omega-3 fatty acid and protein, which aid in promoting healthy scalp and hair growth! In the winter, introduce more oily fruits and vegetables into the diet to counteract dry skin and hair. Step into a healthy diet on the following pages for a good mind, a good body and good hair!

Iron:
- Bolsters hair growth
  - Meat, shellfish, fortified grains and leafy greens

Protein:
- Building block of hair
  - Lean cuts of meat, mix light meat with dark, seafood

Vitamins:
- Metabolic processes
- Biotin
  - Brewer's yeast, nutritional yeast, liver, cauliflower, salmon, bananas, carrots, egg yolks, sardines, legumes and mushrooms
- B6&B12
  - whole grains, oatmeal, skim milk, low fat cheese, eggs, salmon, nuts, nut butters
- Zinc-
  - Shine, lubricates follicles
  - Brightly colored fruits and veggies like strawberries and kiwi, raspberries, mangoes, oranges, red bell peppers
- Vitamin A
  - Apples, apricots, sweet potatoes

Antioxidants:
- Prevents cellular damage
- Healthy scalp and follicular regeneration
  - Herbs, dark chocolate, fresh berries

Sample Breakfast:

Make the first meal rich in biotin and protein, hair's primary components.
• Option 1: Whole-grain tortilla [BIOTIN] with 1 slice lowfat cheese [BIOTIN]; 2 scrambled eggs [BIOTIN]; 3 slices mango
  • Option 2: 1 cup oatmeal [BIOTIN] with skim milk [BIOTIN] and a small handful of walnuts [BIOTIN] and dried apricots; 1/2 grapefruit

Sample Lunch:

Munch on foods containing growth-promoting iron midday.
• Option 1: 3 oz roast beef [IRON] or turkey [IRON] on whole-wheat toast [IRON] with 1 slice lowfat cheese and

1/2 avocado (instead of mayo)
- Option 2: 3 oz grilled chicken breast; small baked sweet potato; salad of 4 cups romaine [IRON], 1/2 cup each

- red bell pepper and chickpeas; 1 tablespoon of olive oil and lemon juice to taste

Sample Snack:

Antioxidant-rich bites between meals make for a healthy scalp.
- Option 1: 1/2 cup unsalted edamame [ANTIOXIDANTS] sprinkled with chili powder
  - Option 2: 1 oz dark chocolate [ANTIOXIDANTS]; 1/2 cup raspberries [ANTIOXIDANTS AND BIOTIN]

Sample Dinner:

Protein for final meal boosts hair and energy levels.
- Option 1: 2 1/2 cups veggie chili consisting of 1/2 cup each red kidney beans [PROTEIN], carrots, potato, peas [PROTEIN] and tomatoes
  - Option 2: 6 oz grilled wild salmon [PROTEIN AND BIOTIN] or steak [PROTEIN]; a salad of 4 cups spinach, 1/2 cup orange slices, 1 oz goat cheese, a handful each of pumpkin seeds and raisins; 1 tbsp olive oil and lemon juice to tast

Step into a healthy diet for a good mind, a good body and good hair!

Hair Color

The topic of hair coloring is controversial. Traditional hair coloring products have ingredients that are carcinogens associated with bladder, breast and other cancers, among hair care professions and clients. In one study released in 2005, the risk increased with more prolonged exposure to darker, more concentrated, permanent dyes. There are other ailments associated with the chemicals in hair dyes, but what is most disturbing is that women using hair dyes risk getting brain cancer passing this risk onto their children, increasing their chances of being born with brain cancer[10].

Let's think a moment about how hair dyes work:

1. Ammonia opens the hair cuticle to allow for the hydrogen peroxide to penetrate the cuticle.
2. The hydrogen peroxide removes the original hair color.
3. Peroxide breaks the chemical bonds in the hair, releasing sulfur.
4. The hydrogen peroxide removes the original hair color.
5. The new permanent color is released into the hair shaft.
6. A silicone based conditioner closes and seals the cuticle.

Hydrogen peroxide, sulfur and ammonia are well-known respiratory track irritants that can cause asthma or a severe allergic reaction. Then, pigment chemicals penetrate the skin and enter the bloodstream. Check the following hair color ingredients, because there is no such thing as a safe chemical hair color. Vanity should not precede health. The bladder, breasts, lungs, immune and endocrine system will thank you! For the best lock care, if commercial coloring is preferred, be careful to implement deep conditioning treatments throughout the year and only color, at the maximum twice a year.

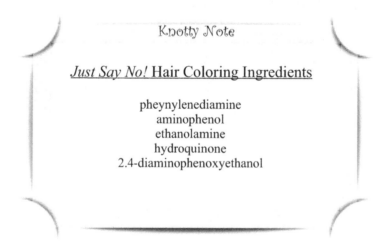

Knotty Note

Just Say No! Hair Coloring Ingredients

pheynylenediamine
aminophenol
ethanolamine
hydroquinone
2.4-diaminophenoxyethanol

---

[10]McCall *et al.* 2005

Green/natural alternatives to synthetic dyes are henna, found in protein conditioners such as: red henna (*Lawsonia inermis, Lawsonia alba, and Lawsonia spinosa*), neutral henna (*Lyzifus spina christi*), and black henna (*Indigofera tinctora*). The colors can be blended for color variation with the addition of indigo and iron oxides. The neutral henna can be added to shampoos and conditioners for conditioning benefits without coloring. The disadvantage of henna is the messy application and its ability to only change the hair color temporarily making it a semi-permanent application. Given that it is a healthy alternative to synthetic dyes and the only colorant with safety approval from the FDA, it's worth the investment. Henna is not recommended if permanent hair dye is in the hair. Other benefits of henna on highly texture hair (or not) is its straightening affect on the hair, increased volume, scalp irritation, increased manageability and attack on dandruff! There are other online resources for color, such as TheHairShebang http://www.etsy.com/shop/thehairshebang? etsy.com that specializes in henna bars that are melted down and combined with nourishing oils to color the hair uniquely. High quality henna is a bright green and sifted many times. Cheaper hennas need sifting, to prevent applicator clogging, or residue left behind in the locks which can lead to damage months later. Never use henna that is bright green and fades to light brown, as it loses potency. Companies may use green henna to make it appear fresher. Some store bought henna has heavy metals that may react in the hair and on the scalp. Safe henna is body art quality henna, such as Karishma brand, which can be mixed with hot coffee or red zinger for a beautiful brown, reddish color. Jamila is another high quality, bridal henna that is super sifted. It can turn gray hairs coppery orange and dark, brown hair an auburn/burgundy tinge in the sun.

Coloring Tips:

Lighten the hair: Treatment shampoos and conditioners with lemon, chamomile, sunflower, calendula

Brighten red hair: Neutral or golden henna in the hair care regimen

Darken the hair: Black walnut, black tea, coffee and licorice root added to conditioners

Transitioning to henna can be overwhelming, the preceding tips should help. Remember, henna can be added to a favorite conditioner or shampoo.

Types and Names of Henna		
RED HENNA	BLACK HENNA	NEUTRAL HENNA
Lawsonia inermis	Indigofera tinctora	Lyzifus spina christi
Lawsonia alba		
Lawsonia spinosa		

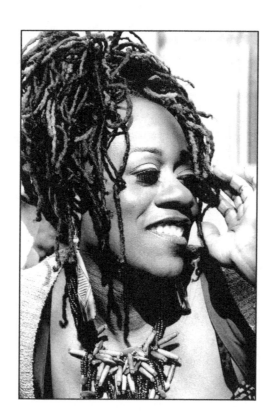

The following rinses can be used to achieve the desired color, slowly. Applicator bottles or old plastic water bottles that can be squeezed come in use when applying a rinse. After washing the hair, towel dry, squeeze out any excessive moisture, before applying the rinse. Then proceed styling locks as usual.

Natural Hair Coloring Recipes

Chamomile Tea Leave-In Rinse

To lighten dark hair with golden highlights with red hue

3 tea bags chamomile tea for a 1/2 cup serving
1/2 cup Aloe Vera gel
1 tbspn warm honey
1 tbspn lemon juice

Tip: Cool, mix and apply with applicator bottle .
Rinses can be stored in a spritz applicator for refresher throughout the week. If storing, make sure to refrigerate and add an essential oil, vitamin E or pinch of vitamin C to preserve the solution.

Chocolate Brunette Hair Pre-Shampoo Rinse

To darken hair

5 tbspn dark roast ground coffee
1 oz black chocolate
2 cups purified water

Boil the ground coffee in 2 cups of water in a shallow pan for 10 min
Add chocolate while coffee is hot
Let the mixture cool

Tip: Mix and apply with applicator bottle .
Rinses can be stored in a spritz applicator for refresher throughout the week. If storing, make sure to refrigerate and add an essential oil, vitamin E or pinch of vitamin C to preserve the solution.

Red Hair Shine Enhancer Pre-Shampoo Rinse

To enhance red hair

1/2 cup beet juice
1/2 cup carrot juice
1/2 cup lemon juice

Mix ingredients, apply to hair, cover and wait
Add a hot towel to accelerate heating
Rinse, Shampoo

Tip: Mix and apply with applicator bottle .

Beat That Dandruff and Lighten the Hair
To lighten hair with golden highlights and counter dandruff

1 cup Neutral henna
1 cup Aloe Vera juice
1 cup lemon juice

Blend in equal proportions, massage into hair and scalp, wait[11] rinse out

Tip: Mix and apply with applicator bottle .
Rinses can be stored in a spritz applicator for refresher throughout the week. If storing, make sure to refrigerate and add an essential oil, vitamin E or pinch of vitamin C to preserve the solution.

Edible hair care is an experience that is out of this world and great for every type of hair! Will locks thrive without implementing healthy hair options? Absolutely! However, remember, holistic care of the body begins with awareness and making conscious choices on what we put in and on our bodies.

---

[11]Apple cider vinegar can replace the lemon juice to keep dark hair dark.

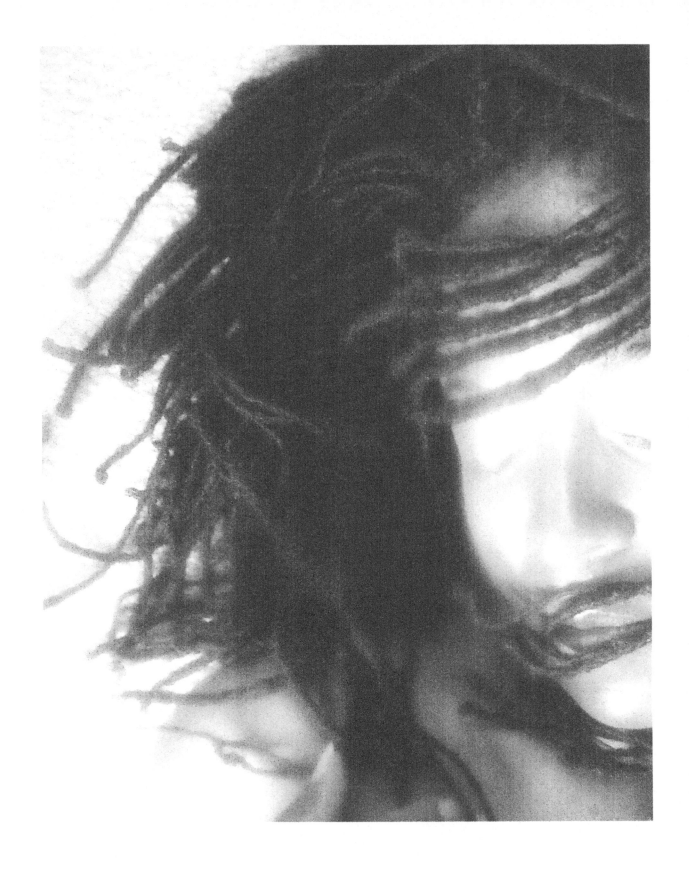

CREATING BEAUTIFUL LOCKS ON A DIME!

The State
of
The
Hair

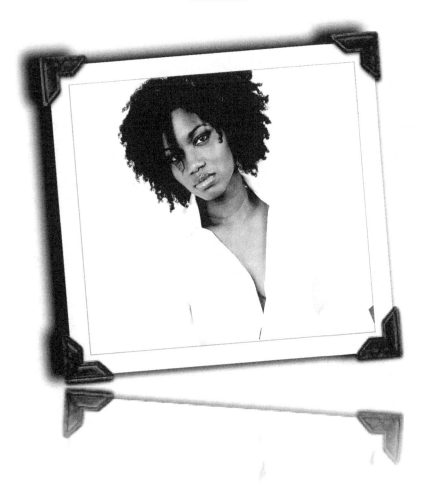

Two Things to Know Before Locking It Down
ok, maybe more

Before the first lock is installed, it's important to understand the state of the hair. Deciding which foundation to begin locks with can be difficult. Instead of getting overwhelmed, the decision can be streamlined by focusing on two key points:

1. Biological Traits of the Hair
2. Health of the Hair

Biological Traits

1. *Density of hair (diameter of the hair shaft)*
2. *Density of hair follicles*
3. *Follicle shape*
4. *Hair texture*
5. *Length of the hair*

Locks can be started by different variations of braids, twists, coils, free-formed or other design foundations. At the end of the day, the foundation will not matter. The importance of the foundation is to find one that works with the natural hair texture, allowing it to remain stationary with minimal movement. The key to how the locks will form is the installation foundation and the tightening technique chosen. Other than these two actions, the hair is in control, not the locker. The installation and maintenance preferences are the two things the locker can participate in as the lock forms, as the hair teaches the locker lessons on patience, endurance and self-esteem that could never be learned in a classroom or in a book.

When deciding which lock foundation to implement, hair density, texture, and health are key factors. Assessing the locker's DNA (deoxyribonucleic acid) instructions determines whether the hair will develop straight or curly, because it is the genetic template that tells each individual cell in the body what to do. The DNA stores the genetic information responsible for everything from body size, height, shape, color and hair texture. This information is stored in the form of amino acids which form a specific pattern, forming the genetic building blocks that dictate messages to the cell, giving direction and order. These building blocks are known as amino acids and are found in the form of Adenine, Thymine, Guanine, and Cytosine, in the hair, forming specific codes that determine hair texture. The DNA is also responsible for the actual length of the hair, translating hormones in the body that control DNA replication in the life cycle of a hair follicle! DNA traits are passed down from parents through the family genes manifesting in the hair texture.

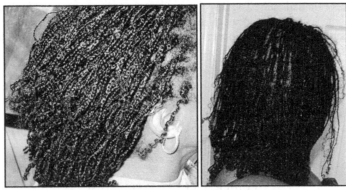
Thick follicles, minimal spacing versus thin follicles

Density

The density of the hair strand (diameter of the hair strand/shaft) and density of the follicles on the scalp (distance between the follicles) influence hair behavior as well. For example, when considering the thickness of the hair, follicles can be spaced apart or densely packed together naturally. Those with "thin" hair are known to have a lower density of follicles/square inch on the scalp, as opposed to those with a high number of follicles/square inch have thick hair, the scalp is usually not visible between partings. Those with a small hair diameter can have thin hair, as well.

The density of the hair on the scalp is important because density of the hair follicles and diameter of the hair strand impact the size of the lock. If the locker has "thin hair," it could be from one of two things. As mentioned, when the density of the hair follicles is sparse, there is a lot of scalp that is naturally visible and the hair appears thin. This could be a result of age, because an older adult may have a different hair density on the scalp, than s/he had as a child, as the skin on the scalp becomes less taut, the scalp loses its collagen over time, the follicle distance widens and the hair appears thin. In this case, the true texture doesn't change, the arrangement of the follicles on the scalp changes. The thickness/diameter of a hair strand impacts hair behavior, as well. Density of the hair strand diameter may also influence lock thickness upon installation. If the density of the strand is small, the lock shaft's diameter can be thin, resulting in the appearance of thin locks. The larger the diameter, the larger the lock can swell, as the individual hair strands swell within the lock. The amount gathered for the locking section is dependent upon the density of the hair follicles and density of the hair strand. This trait also impacts how ingredients react with the hair texture, as well as styling options[12].

Density of the hair strand is independent of density of the scalp; however, when the two are found on the same head, they can impact the hair's appearance within the mature lock. For example, newly installed Sisterlocks™ are thinner and stiffer than normal, and look like tiny braids. The locks will thicken and fill over time, with a couple of shampoos, as the natural texture begins to express itself[13]. New locks usually show a lot of scalp in the newborn phase and at tightening time, accentuating the density. If a locker's 'thin' hair is a concern, it's important to note that the hair will gradually fill in over time. Patience is required. The locker can just opt for the backcombed, free-formed locks, twisted or coiled installations which expand quickly allowing the hair to frizz, minimizing the

---

[12]The Holistic Hair Care Chapter

[13]Cornwell, Joanne. That Hair Thing. 2nd Edition ed. San Diego: Sisterlocks Pub, 2009. Print.

appearance of scalp. For a full look, these traditional foundations swell, giving a thicker appearance, adding to the hair's volume and thickness, immediately. The density of the hair on the scalp can help determine what type of locks the locker will prefer. Some locks will appear full, giving the hair a thicker appearance within a week following installation. Varying densities are why many lockers can install the same foundation; yet, have very different results upon maturity.

Knotty Note

Test 1

Follicle Density: Scalp Test

Visually examine a section of scalp per square inch on the scalp.

1. Notice the space on the scalp between two plaits from forehead to nape of the neck. The spacing will determine if hair texture is thin, medium or thick.
2. Take note of the spacing in various sections on the scalp and compare distance between follicles.
3. A distance larger than a centimeter, will express as thin hair. With follicles closer, the hair will generally be thicker.

Knotty Note

Test 2

Hair Strand Density Test

Visually examine a strand of hair.

1. Fine, thin hair is almost translucent and feels like silk when rolled between thumb and second finger.
2. Medium hair is easier to see, feels like cotton when rolled between thumb and second finger.
3. Thick hair is coarse to touch, feels like wool when rolled between thumb and finger, makes a noise, when rolled between thumb and second finger.

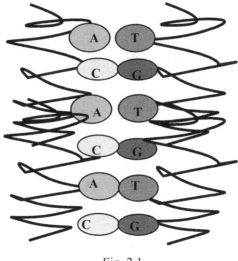

Fig. 2.1
DNA

Follicles & Textures

The anatomy of the hair is important for the at home maintenance and health of maturing locks. The hair is made of two major parts: the shaft and the root. The shaft is the hair that grows above the skin, which is dead. The root grows below the skin, inside of the follicle. For the purpose of applying a secure lock foundation, the shape and direction of the hair follicle shapes the hair texture; and, therefore influences the future lock. The shape and direction of the living follicle are important because the position of the follicles along the scalp help to determine the shape of the emerging hair strand. According to Andre Walker, the developer of a well-recognized hair typing system based upon follicle shape, there are four main hair texture categories[14]:

Type 1- Straight Hair: The follicles are parallel to the surface of the scalp; therefore, the hair emerges straight from the scalp, forming a straight hair shaft. Ninety percent cuticle due to the hard keratin (rope-like protein filaments throughout the hair strand that provide structure) protein layer. Thick cuticle made of twelve to fifteen protective layers, thin cortex, no medulla. This hair texture resists locking.

---

[14]Google for more information

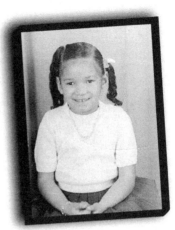

Type 2-Wavy hair follicles form from a slight bend of the hair follicle, causing the hair to emerge from the scalp with a slight angle, curving the hair strand. Wavy hair has a thick cuticle, thin cortex, sparse medulla. Hair resists locking.

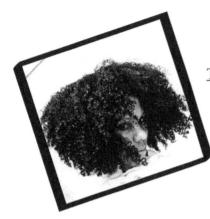

Type 3-Curly, wavy hair results from a higher bend of the hair follicle, which puts the follicle slightly perpendicular to the scalp, causing a winding formation of the hair strand as it emerges from the scalp. Type 3 texture is 85% cortex. Curly hair has a thicker cortex, thin cuticle with more keratin content than Type 4 hair, partial medulla. Hair locks with some assistance.

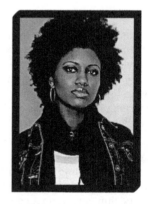

Type 4-Kinky hair forms from the perpendicular position of the follicle to the scalp, causing the hair strand to emerge from the follicle, bending at a right angle and continuing to form as a sharp coil as the hair constantly emerges from the scalp. Thin cuticle is made of only 4-7 layers of keratin. Many textures may be present on the scalp ranging from Type 3-4[15]. With a thick cortex, almost 90% of hair composition, medulla present. Hair easily locks on its own.

Follicles are the only living portion of the hair, and are extremely important. The hair is made of a shaft and a root. The hair root/papilla grows below the skin, inside of the follicle (Fig. 2.2). Feed the follicles, and a healthy head of hair will grow from the root and medulla if the hair is highly textured! The health of the hair lies within this important compartment and feeding it daily is important. The DNA directs the hair follicle's shape and direction of each hair strand. The wider and more parallel the follicle shape, to the surface, the straighter the hair. The more perpendicular to the scalp and narrow the follicle (Type 4), the curlier and highly textured the hair.

---

[15]Hair textures can be further designated by a,b,c: a-stands for the straightest hair texture, c-the tightest curl texture.

Hair can range from Type 1 straight hair to Type 4. Type 4 hair can be well-defined pencil thin corkscrew curls, kinky or wiry and brittle or puff up in a cloud of napps that are undefined and C-Napps as defined by the various blogs on the net[16].

Type 4 hair that is left alone will eventually mat into locks. Type 2 and 3 are keratin rich, with thicker cuticles than Type 4 hair, and behave differently. These textures will lock best with manipulation and effort. Type 4, highly textured hair, is uniquely diverse and usually a melting pot of many textures, instead of one uniform texture, but winds into a tight curl. Installing a lock that works to secure the straight pattern is critical to prevent slippage and unwinding of the lock, to help shape the direction of the future lock and help stabilize the lock. If a lock is installed by coils and palm-rolled into a head of Type 2 or Type 3 hair, the hair will constantly unravel making it difficult to wash, style and keep the lock pattern. However, if this grade of hair is installed into some type of 3-step combination method[17], stable locks can develop easily.

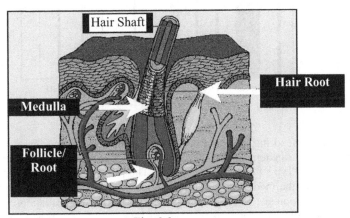

Fig. 2.3
Hair follicle and shaft

Length

Each hair strand undergoes a cycle of growth, while in the follicle. The first phase, the anagen phase, is the hair growth phase and lasts 2-6 years. During this phase, the papilla is attached to the base of the hair shaft, thriving and growing, producing the protein keratin. On average, in a hundred days, an inch of the hair will emerge from the papilla, during this phase. The next phase is the catagen phase which is a resting phase for the hair. There is no growth during this stage; and, the hair strand undergoes a period of inactivity for two to three weeks as the hair follicle shrinks. The next phase is the telogen phase. The new epithelial skin layer forms, pushing the layer up and out, making room for new hair. The papilla is an important feature of the hair strand because it is fed by tiny blood vessels that feed the hair strand nutrients, taking away waste. The papilla is visible when the hair sheds during the telogen phase, falling into the matrix of the lock. The papilla releases from the follicle and is pushed out from the

[16]http://www.nappyme.wordpress.com

[17]See The Root of the Matter Chapter

scalp[18]. The direction, shape and health of the hair follicle determine the form of the emerging hair strand, forming a terminal number of hair follicles on the scalp at birth, roughly 100,000.

The follicle constantly goes through cycles of growth and rest that will impact the health of the hair strands, lasting in cycles of up to roughly five years of growth and replacement. Approximately 100 hairs a day are lost for natural reasons. If there is any concern about shedding, inspect the lock. If there is a hair strand attached to a white bulb, it's naturally shed hair. The stages of hair growth are impacted by, hormonal changes, severe emotional stress, nutrition, childbirth, fever, surgery, illness, blood loss, crash diets void of protein, and chemicals in the body such as: NSAIDS, ibuprofen, antidepressants, beta-blockers, birth control pills, retinoids and calcium channel blockers. All of these entities can lead to an excessive loss of hair. When this occurs, the papilla is visible and hair loss can be assessed by the presence of the bulb (papilla) attachment.

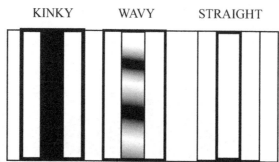

KINKY   WAVY   STRAIGHT

Fig. 2.4 The Cross-section of a medulla in
kinky, wavy and straight hair.

The nutrients from the papilla feed into the core of the hair strand, via the cortex and the medulla, if present. The papilla is also responsible for transferring hair hormones, which regulate and impact the hair growth cycle. The medulla (Fig. 2.4) is present in Type 4 hair, but not others. The medulla houses the melanocytes, hair color cells, in Type 4 hair. The theory is that the medulla is linked to temperature regulation as a sensor that helps to lower body temperature in cultures from tropical climates while giving the hair structural support. The melanocytes are in the cortex in Type 1, 2, 3 hair strands. The cortex is the layer that takes up most of the hair strand in highly textured hair by 85-90%! The cortex houses the disulfide bonds, responsible for holding the coil in highly textured hair. It also holds the proteins, amino acids and hydrogen bonds, which impact the elasticity, resulting in expansion and contraction of the hair. As a result, the diameter of highly textured hair is much larger than straight hair and the behavior of highly textured hair mimics the large cortex composition by conforming to various shapes and lengths. Highly textured hair can be molded and reshaped because the cuticle is thin, allowing for bends in the hair. There's a lot of nutrition that is vital to the health of a hair strand in this core matrix. This cortex matrix is protected by cuticle cells that form the outer, protective layer of the hair strand. The cuticle only composes 10-15% or 4-7 layers in highly textured hair, versus 12-15 in Type 1, straight hair. As a result, straight hair is more challenging to lock because of its high composition of keratin- rich cuticle. The hard keratin protein is firm, straight and not easily stretched.

Known as coarse, highly textured-Type 4 hair is actually extremely fragile, *not* coarse. The cuticle cell layers, scaled together, must keep all of the nutrients inside of the hair strand. With only 10% composition, it's a difficult job for a cuticle to protect highly textured hair. Environment, manipulation, styling habits, nutrition, and general maintenance work consistently against the force of the cuticle, often resulting in damage, as the cuticle opens via a split or a tear, compromising the health of the hair strand. Protein conditioners that are said to "reseal" the cuticle are only

---

[18]Whenever a white tip is visually seen attached to a hair strand, the hair strand has shed. Please be aware that a traumatic experience such as surgery, child birth etc., can cause hair to become dormant and shed for up to six months as chemicals leave the body. It's not uncommon to see a lot of hair bulbs/papilla 6-12 months post surgery as the chemicals are shedding the terminal residue from the body for up to a year!

temporary and require constant reapplication. The only thing that can resolve a damaged cuticle is trimming away the damage. The benefit of locking highly textured hair is to protect the cuticles as strands of hair combine to form a protective chord against these forces.

A final consideration is scab hair. Scab hair is hair that has usually been damaged from straightening by a hot comb or chemical process. Scab hair occurs when a previously damaged follicle regenerates hair. The hair that emerges, loses its original tightly coiled texture and is unnaturally straight. Typically, it's straighter, thinner, exhibits less vitality and weaker than the original texture. Scab hair may or may not return to its virgin hair texture because the bonds have been irreparably damaged, usually via a hot appliance or a chemical. When the follicles are damaged from the concomitant use of a straightening device, along with petroleum or mineral oil, scab hair can occur. If product seeps down into the follicles of the scalp, the follicles can become damaged, altering the texture of the hair. The follicle can be so damaged that it stops generating hair permanently. If scab hair is semi-permanent, it can take from six months to a year of no chemical application for the hair to return to its original formation. Combination-installation techniques can be implemented to circumvent this damage for scab hair to lock.

How to Decide which locks work for your Hair Texture!

Straight No Chaser
Locking Straight Hair

Type 1, Type 2 and some Type 3 hair textures are challenging to lock; however, it is possible. These hair textures may resist curling and matting. Because these three hair textures predominately consists of protein rich keratin in the outer core, they exhibit cuticle behaviors, lying straight, and resistant to locking. This texture does not naturally form a tight coil, inhibiting the matrix from intertwining and forming a net of shed hair. The coils that are necessary for locks to mature naturally are absent in straight hair, and wavy hair; therefore, straight hair must be intentionally locked and matted to force the hair to mature into locks. When considering which foundation to install for Type 1, 2 or 3, factor in a combination install method to create a meshwork of hair that mats, forming a stable foundation to build a lock upon. Setting the hair into a locked pattern that will minimize movement, unraveling and frizzing is vital or the hair will not lock. Because locking the foundation is the most difficult step in this process, personality, preference and lifestyle will have to take the back burner, as much patience is required for the lock transformation to occur. Care must be taken with hair textures Typed 1, 2 and 3, especially when the hair needs to be washed and manipulated. Using a 3-step combination method such as latching/braiding/twisting first, followed up with the second step, backcombing, to lock the hair in place, then a palm-roll is the best way to secure a lock with a straight hair texture. A forced foundation made by integrating a combination technique is best because straighter hair must be manipulated in order to mat and form locks.

Backcombing is the primary method used to lock straight hair. Backcombing, teasing the hair from the ends of the hair towards the scalp manually, incrementally down the length of the hair shaft, while integrating a 3-step combination method, encourages hair to lock as the hair mats and tangles when teased. Backcombing can also be used independently of of the first step, by simply backcombing the hair, then palm-rolling to set. Setting the foundation with braids, twists or latched locks will further enhance the integrity of the lock, keeping the hair together. The hair length must be one to two inches at installation[19].

---

[19]If locking straight hair, hair resistant to locking, install the foundation first. The second step, backcombing, will further secure the lock. The third step, palm-rolling will help shape the lock. Disclaimer: Any texture hair can be started with a variety of lock methods. The methods suggested are the easiest methods to lock hair based upon texture. Backcombing can be done with or without the additional preliminary step of braids/twists/latched hair; however, if the hair is extra resistant, it is a complementary step that can help to lock in the foundation.

Curly and Tight is Alright!

For those with Type 3-4 type hair

Like straight hair, the key consideration for locking Type 4 hair is the varying degrees of textures within the head and length. Unlike straight hair, length is a pertinent consideration with highly textured hair. Length matters with straight hair; however, regardless of length, straight hair is best installed with a 3-step combination method, requiring one-two inches of length minimum to start. There are many options for the highly textured locker that depend secondly on length. Highly textured hair begins in the Type 3 range. Some Type 3 textures can be wound tightly and found in a head of tightly coiled Type 4 hair. It is rare for one head of highly textured hair to have only one type of texture, it's usually a mixture of many. The challenge is choosing a foundation that will secure the forming lock and prevent unraveling. Because of the inherent biological characteristics of this hair texture, this hair will coil, wave, twist and turn. The key for a successful head of locks is to lock the texture patch, not the full head of hair! By focusing on the texture in each patch of hair, applying a foundation that will resist unraveling will accelerate the locking process by preventing movement of the hair. A straight, wavy texture may need a tighter foundation that resists unraveling, encouraging the locking process. If the locks are initiated with a uniform foundation over the entire head, using the various techniques applicable to the hair texture encourages hair to mobilize.

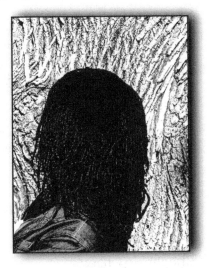

Unlike straight hair textures, highly textured hair easily locks versus any other texture. The characteristic coil and spiral configuration result in shrinkage, easily contributing to the matting process. In addition, the unique coil formation is like melanin in dark skin. Melanin absorbs the energy of light the same as the springs of the hair coils absorb energy for motion. This manifests the physical principal of kinetic energy and potential energy. According to Wiki, potential energy is energy stored within a physical system as a result of the position or configuration of the different parts of that system, in this case, the highly textured hair. The helical formation of highly textured hair stores this energy in the form of spiral bonds bound by a unique formation of the amino acid bases within the cortex of the hair strand. Because of this formation, the hair can transmit (elasticity) and store energy (shrinkage): the hair will transmit energy if the hair is released, or store energy if the hair is left alone. The unique spiral formation fairs better when left uncombed, due to its fragile and powerful energy bearing characteristics. This formation is frequently recognized in the helical formation of a DNA strand, the shape of a tornado, the form of a slinky toy, the unique shape of a strand of hair with a texture that ranges from bouncy curls, intricate coils to hard zig zags of Type 4 textures. All uniquely individual; yet, bearing the ability to hold and release energy. This hair texture was made to lock and prefers styles that protect the hair, encouraging growth and vitality.

The first question to answer when locking highly textured hair is what texture is the hair. The ability of the hair to lock is dependent upon the texture of the hair. Are the bends sharp with jagged, fragile edges, straight, wavy with a bouncy curl or a head full of tight, pencil sized spiral coils? Having a working knowledge of the type of coil, bend, and texture will allow the locker to choose a locking pattern that can lock in the various hair textures, reduce movement, and allow the hair to lock. In fact, simply leaving Type 4 texture alone, will lead to matting, and eventually locks. As a result, some Type 3 and all Type 4 hair will reasonably lock on their own, without manipulation, resulting in free-formed or organic locks.

Because of pattern variability on a single head of hair, texture must be assessed on a section by section basis. It is important to work with the hair texture at that given location, rather than making a patch of hair conform to a uniform design. For example, the front of the head may have a straight, wavy hair pattern, the back of the head may be tightly curled, the sides may do something in between and the middle of the head may be coarse and unruly. The highly textured hair may install and hold well with braids, twists, coils but the straight, wavy hair may need a variation of latched locks, backcombing and palm-rolling. Combining a few techniques to eventually get the hair to lock will not disturb the lock transformation process. Locks are uniquely imperfect and non-uniform. If ignored, a hair that is locked into a pattern that does not work to secure the texture of the hair will unravel, bunch and slip. On the contrary, the appropriate locked pattern will reward the locker with a crown of locks with minimal drama.

Locking techniques have advanced and are no longer relegated to chemically free hair; however, it is best to begin with virgin, chemical free hair, when installing traditional locks. This philosophy is shared among the grass roots natural hair movement[20]. Hair that is processed with chemicals is inherently weak because the sulfide bonds responsible for the curl of the hair have been altered and broken, exposing the core of the hair strand pulp to dryness and moisture depletion. Moisture is released as the bonds are damaged to allow for the straightening process to occur. If a lock is built with this foundation at the root, it could compromise the health of the future lock. For the most successful journey, it's important that the locker grows chemically free hair first and spends the necessary time becoming acquainted with the unique characteristics of highly textured hair, such as density, elasticity, shrinkage, and texture of the hair. The core of the lock lays a foundation; and it's best that that foundation is fortified with strong disulfide and hydrogen bonds that can catch the hair that will fall into the lock, forming the inner-core matrix, which is paramount to the growth of a healthy lock.

Some lockers will transition from a chemical perm straight to locks; however, the most successful lockers take more time to get acquainted with their hair. Through a poll conducted on www.nappturality.com[21] *April, 2010*: 9 out of 10 pollsters agree that those who took time to know their natural hair texture for a few years before locking versus those that went straight from the big cut, cutting off all the chemically relaxed hair from the virgin hair, to locks, were more likely to never cut away their locks. Those who transitioned with a chemical relaxer straight to locks, often cut their locks off after three or four years to experience loose hair. When a locker has experienced the frustration of multiple hour long sessions of detangling and styling, product and style frustration, s/he is more apt to appreciate the simplicity of locks and the ease of styling with nary an inclination to revert and remove the locks. This lesson is only learned by spending time with loose-chemical-free hair.

Another consideration is the length of the hair. Length, be it long or short, is no longer an obstacle in the locking process. Lockers with at least half of an inch of new growth can have locks installed which sponge applicators that create dreadlocks in a circular motion, now. In fact, the shorter the hair the better! When used, only half of an inch of highly textured hair is needed to start locks[22]. Hair longer than one inch would require assistance. Because of advances, locks can be started on all textures and lengths! Comb coils, and two stranded twists can be installed with at least half of an inch of hair; however, they can quickly unravel for lengths longer than an inch. Some other well known techniques to start locks for short hair with the same effect by rubbing the hair with a wet wash cloth, brushing damp hair in a circular motion or installing coils with a rat-tailed comb or fingers.

Braids, Interlocks, Sisterlocks™/Brotherlocks™ and strand twists are excellent foundations to begin with long highly textured hair, because they will hold the hair in a tight pattern. Long hair takes the longest amount of time to transform into locks, because the length of the hair is compromised for at least a year and a half, as the locks transform. Growth will appear to come to a halt, as the locks transform methodically from the inside out. It is a long process and the transformation takes time and energy. When short hair transforms into locks, length is noticeable more quickly than locking from long hair. Short hair will begin to look like locks within one to two months. When locking long hair, remember that the goal is to minimize movement so the hair can lock and the preceding methods achieve that goal.

---

[20]There is a debate that hair cannot be locked from chemically processed hair. It can. The real issue is the health of the lock, which must be the first priority. Health over vanity must come first. Always try to lock from chemically free/virgin hair if at all possible.

[21]www.nappturality.com

[22]Sites like www.nudred.com will show an applicator used to create dreadlocks.

Hair Health
Elasticity,

Note the hair texture in the lock chart. The hair health will determine how the hair will lock. There are physical tests that can be applied to test the biological traits and health of the hair, that are independent of hair texture. Hair health is impacted by porosity and elasticity. Porosity is the ability of hair to hold water. Porosity is a consideration, because the easier the hair mats, the quicker it will lock as the cuticles are lifted, open and more prone to snagging and sticking. A highly porous texture will begin locking quickly. Elasticity is a measure of how long the hair will stretch, while retaining it's original shape upon release. Note the various hair health indicators:

Knotty Note

Test 3

The Slide Test: Porosity

The amount of moisture the hair can hold, the more porous the hair. The more porous the hair, the more easily it mats. Porous hair is porous because of the raised cuticles. Raised cuticles influence the amount of liquid that can penetrate the hair. It's important to assess the health of the cuticle. Hair can be porous from physical or chemical damage. Advise on healthy treatments inside and out to restore hair health.

Test 1:
Lift the hair from the scalp with one hand.
Push the hair strands downward toward the scalp with the other hand.

Result: If there's lot of drag the hair is porous
Smooth hair is most likely not porous
- Very porous: hair tangles easily
- Normal: hair tangles slightly
- Resistant: hair refuses to tangle

Test 4

The Roll Test: Porosity

Test 2:
Wet a portion of the hair

Result:
Resistant-water rolls off of this hair, barely getting absorbed. It is known as hair that has poor absorption and it is prone to dryness naturally.
Average -Describes hair with abnormal amount of absorption. This hair is in good condition.
Extreme -Water may roll off of this hair, coupled with poor hair health.
Uneven -A combination of any of the above.

Test 5

Elasticity:5 in 5 test

Purpose: *To determine hair health.*

Test:
Remove 5 strands of hair from the scalp.
Hold them between thumb and index finger.
Pull hair taut for 5 seconds.

Result:
If the hair returns to original curl pattern, it's in good condition.
If it returns only 50% or less, it is structurally weak and needs extra hydration from the inside out and moisture conditioning treatments.

If any of the tests show the hair to be in poor condition, advise client to eat a healthy diet. Additional supplementation of folic acid and drinking half the body weight in water will begin to restore the hair's health. Condition the hair with herbal tea conditioning treatments. Advise the client to practice protective hairstyles. It's very important to not cut blunt ends into the hair before locking. Small braids, stranded twists or extension styles would help, along with daily massages using the healthy nourishing oil and spritzing once a day[23].

---

[23]The Holistic Hair Care Chapter

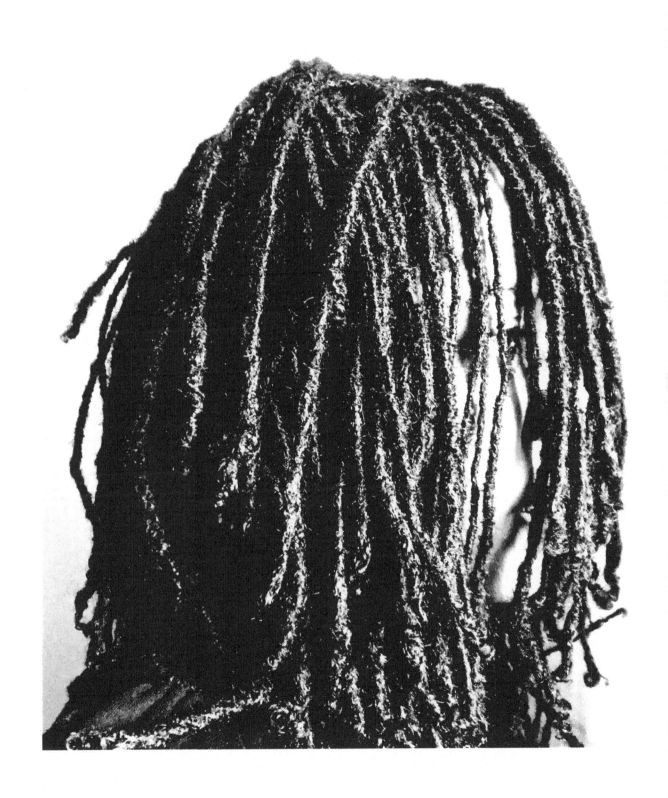

CREATING BEAUTIFUL LOCKS ON A DIME!

3

Now What?
How Do I Find the Right Locks
for Me?
Choosing The Right Locks for Me!

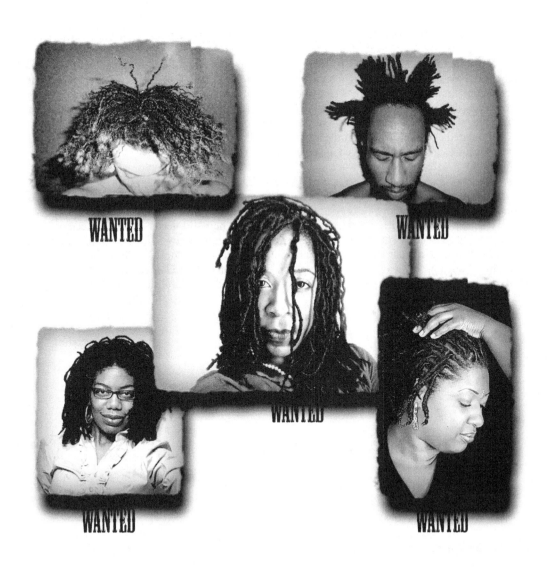

WANTED

WANTED

WANTED

WANTED

WANTED

1. What method should I choose to start my locks?
2. How should I install my locks?
3. How will I maintain my locks?
4. Will I maintain my locks on my own or continue to see a locktician?
5. How do I maintain my locks in between appointments?

Chapter two discussed the importance of factoring in the biological traits and health of hair, when deciding which locking style to install. When guiding the shape of the future lock, practical concerns such as lifestyle and personal preference must be the next step along the lock continuum. Knowing the biological structure and inherent characteristics of the hair are key to growing a healthy head of locks[24]. The foundation of an emerging lock is just a hairstyle, because the foundation does not shape the future lock, rather it serves as a lock anchor, guiding the direction of the future lock-to-be, influencing the lock in subtle ways. The tightening-maintenance technique will determine the shape of the future lock. Locks can be started many different ways; however, one day a lock will naturally look like matted chords of hair, regardless of the installation method chosen. Once the hair is locked, it will stay locked until the locks are manually picked apart, cut off, or taken down[25].

The foundation care will determine the shape of the future lock. One of the many lessons learned along the journey of locking is that the hair rules; and, relinquishing control to the locking process is its own unique mental journey. As a result, one of the worst things any locker can do is to totally ignore the hair. Locks don't need the same type of attention as loose hair; locks have different needs. However, locked hair still needs attention, needing to be watered, fed, cared for, and touched to grow and thrive. The maintenance and care are two vital techniques that can determine the future of a dreaded lock of hair. Deciding which foundation to begin locks with can be difficult. Instead of getting overwhelmed, streamline the decision by the process of elimination, and develop a system that creates a lock journey that is rewarding. The following diagram lists just some of the possibilities to finding the right locks on a dime!

---

[24]The State of the Hair Chapter

[25]The Great Take-Down Chapter

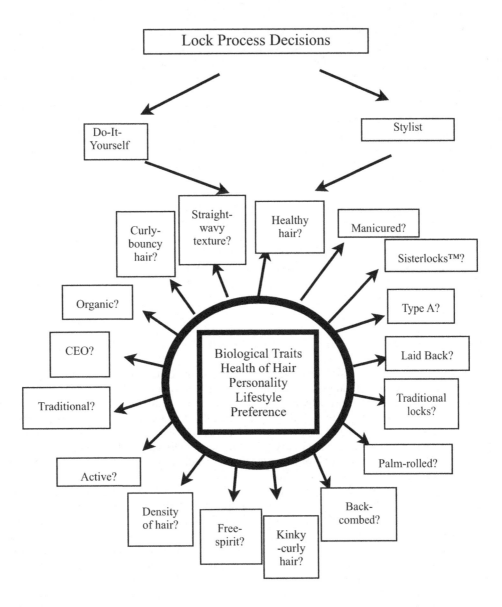

Fig. 3.1 The Locking Process

Use this visual while filling out the lock chart in the index. The decision is yours, be empowered. The following section should help to sort it all out.

Personality
low maintenance, high maintenance, tightening personality, preference

The new locker has decided that locks would be the perfect hairstyle! That's great! Locking is a wonderful journey of self-actualization and acceptance often evolving into a greater level of self-awareness. However, there are personality considerations vital in the evaluation process for the new locker: personality, stress, behavior, low maintenance, high maintenance, tightening preference and tightening personality. There is a difference in the lock journey between a locker that wants to lock for spiritual and personal reasons versus a new locker that just wants the latest hairstyle. The person that wants to develop and grow with a head of locks may be more committed to the journey and want more out of the journey than just a hairstyle. The time and energy put into a lock foundation of a committed locker can come back as a rich investment of a beautiful garden of locks with flexibility and manageability, years down the road. A locker looking for the latest hair style will settle for lock extensions, such as Geni® locks, to satisfy his/her need, immediately[26]. For example, a person with a high maintenance personality would usually prefer for his/her locks to be maintained by someone else. A high maintenance personality may prefer a set of locks that complement his/her personality requiring pampering and attention. Pampering could be important to this personality and a do-it-yourself option is only an option if necessary. The new locker may develop a love for the locks and keep them over the long term-but the personality of a locker who prefers to have an immediate hairstyle need not be as labor intensive as the personality of a locker who wants to understand and enjoy the intricacies of the locking process.

It is important to assess the locker's personality. Does the new locker have a controlling, low key, passive, aggressive, passive-aggressive, independent, dependent personality? Perhaps the new locker has a high degree of self-confidence and could care less about the challenging early weeks of locking that others associate with drama and dislike. Fig. 3.2 summarizes a general overview of the lock foundation and key personality traits. It's key to match a lock foundation with the proper personality because a person with a controlling personality would not fair well with organic, free-formed locks that grow at will; neither would a free spirit fair well with manicured locks that require monthly visits.

Lifestyle
Work environment, support network, activity level, religious beliefs

Because lifestyle, work environment and peer influence can encompass the majority of the day. A person's daily routine and lifestyle is a vital consideration when deciding the lock foundation and tightening method to implement. Does the new locker have a strong support network? When co-workers, family and friends begin to chastise, or say unkind words about the unruliness of a new lock foundation, will the new locker have the proper support to make it through the rough days? Does the new locker have a support network that will pour words of love and encouragement while the hair transforms belligerently? Or, will the new locker be challenged from the work place to home with negativity? Workplace rules, like it or not, are a real consideration. Will the policy affect the new locker? If the locker is in the service industry, sales or senior leadership, will it present challenges or obstacles? Does the new-locker have a high level of physical activity from exercise or sports? Once again, a high level of physical activity can translate into manipulation of the hair. For example, there are rules in the armed services that prohibit certain natural hairstyles[27]. Considering the new locker's religious beliefs are important as well. For example, Christians may express interest in locking; yet, share that false perceptions that locks are anti-Christian. Women of certain Islamic sects don't allow others to see their hair, this is a consideration. Counseling from a stylist or spiritual guidance on the significance of the locks, will help the locker to determine the best foundation with the total person in mind. Careers that require head gear are also impacted by the locking process. If the locker is impacted by workplace rules, further research and counseling may be necessary to help the new locker find alternatives to circumvent daily challenges.

---

[26]Lock extensions are not discussed in this manual.

[27]AFI 36-2903: Dreadlocks are not authorized.

Tightening Personality

There are three core methods to tighten the roots as the new growth sprouts from the scalp; however, the tightening maintenance should only be performed within a window of every four to six weeks, at the most. This can be a challenge to an individual who expects hair to appear meticulous and groomed all of the time[28]. The key is the time frame. No matter how frizzy and undone the hair becomes, aesthetics must be secondary to the health of the hair, and waiting a full four weeks is a must. This cannot be emphasized enough. The type of foundation and tightening

Combination Lock Installation/Personality Chart		
Type of Lock	Tightening Method	Personality/Lifestyle
Sisterlock™ Brotherlock™ Interlock	interlocked	high maintenance busy schedule active lifestyle athlete reserved detail-oriented
Braids Twists	interlocked free-formed palm-rolled	low key easy going may be low maintenance
Organic Free-formed	usually free-formed	extremely laid back into low maintenance
Back-combed	usually free-formed may be interlocked may be palm-rolled	laid back Low maintenance
Coils	free-formed palm-rolled interlocked	medium maintenance traditional

Fig. 3.2 The best decision is the best decision from the individual. The resource guide in this book
is a template of best practices frequently used within the locked community, at large.

method chosen can and should be symbiotic with the needs of the new locker, for a successful journey. Please take the time to evaluate the personality and evaluate with Fig 3.2 when deciding on the foundation and maintenance, because it will directly correlate to the emotional journey and satisfaction that comes as the locks mature.

---

[28]See The Root of the Matter Chapter.

Case Study

Case Study 1:

Want-to-be locker works for a corporate fortune 500 company. S/he has one to two inches of highly textured hair. The hair is very thick with a large diameter. His/Her hair is a tight Type 4 texture and s/he is an avid marathon runner who sweats and works out a lot. S/he wants to throw caution to the wind and free-form because s/he hates doing hair and loves the look and freedom of growing organic locks. S/he would prefer to 'maintain' his/her own hair and loves the option of self-maintenance, if at all.

Case Study 2:

Want-to-be locker works for a corporate fortune 500 company. S/he has one to two inches of highly textured hair. The hair is very thick with a large diameter. His/Her hair is a tight 4b/c texture and s/he is an avid marathon runner who sweats and works out a lot. S/he is concerned about his/her hair. S/he wants to lock, but wants a method of

CASE I	CASE II
Texture-4	Texture-4
Length 1-2 inches	Length 1-2 inches
Density/scalp-thick	Density/scalp-thick
Density/hair-wide	Density/hair-wide
Personality-free and wild	Personality-reserved, Type A
Preference-DIY	Preference-DIY
braidlocks, free-formed	braidlocks, interlocked

locking that will control the frizzy look as much as possible. If it is at all possible, s/he would like to maintain his/her hair herself, and keep it neat, controlling as much of the process as s/he can, while 'Doing-It-Yourself.' The personality, lifestyle and preference of the two lockers are very different; however, everything else: texture, length, density is the same. Because they have highly textured hair, there are options to suit each locker.

Result

<u>Case I</u> would be a great candidate for organic locks or free-formed locks, because s/he doesn't mind throwing caution to the wind and getting messy. Organic locks require no installation and minimal care. S/he has the boldness to do it and the confidence to rock it at headquarters. Or s/he can choose to free-form, after receiving an install foundation. After installing a foundation, the roots would be left to grow freely with popping only[29], no twisting or latching to tighten.

<u>Case II</u> would be a great candidate for braidlocks, because braids will remain intact for many months, usually, not losing a pattern remains until the end of the first year, or later. Presently, whether in the military or workplace, braids are an acceptable hairstyle, which make it a clever option for concerned parties, with workplace concerns. Braidlocks can be installed by the locker and maintained inexpensively if preferred. Traditional locks are locks that can be maintained by the locker, inexpensively. Sisterlocks™ must be maintained by a certified consultant to officially retain their credentialed name of Sisterlocks™[30]. Take into consideration the following specifications when deciding which foundation works best for the new locker.

---

[29]Semi-free forming occurs when the roots are allowed to grow freely without maintenance to tighten. Popping of the roots may or may not occur.

[30]There is an ongoing debate between those with Sisterlocks™ and other lockers. Deviating from the Sisterlocks training is considered by some to no longer be Sisterlocks™, others differ. The debate continues. Dr Cornwell's book mentions her emphasis on lock integrity. Client training available as well.

Building A Strand-Twist Foundation

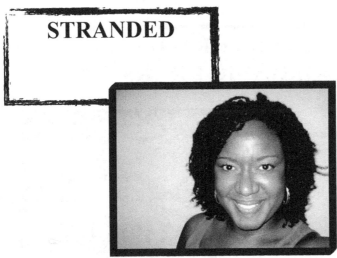

STRANDED

2-Strand Twist
$$

Personality:
• Patient, accepting personality
• May want periodic maintenance
• May prefer self-maintenance
• Concerned about thin hair, will begin to expand and frizz quickly

Hair Texture:
• Type 4
• Type 1,2,3, twists may be step 1 in a 3-step combination method[31]

Advantage:
- If a full look is desired for a thin haired locker, this style will swell and frizz quickly, giving a full appearance.
- Can be used in 3-step combination, as the first step, backcombing as the second step, palm-rolling the third step
- Pattern will disappear quickly, totally between months 6-12 for most lockers
- Can easily be self-maintained
- Lock size can be controlled
- 2-4 inches of hair to install at a minimum

Disadvantage:
- Easily unravels, lots of frizz and shrinkage
- Military does not permit dreadlocks[32]
- Societal perceptions as hair transforms into locks

Types of Twists:

Senegalese Twists
Riqui
2-Strand
3-Strand
Twisty Locks
Twist Extensions

---

[31] Three-step combination method: First step binds the hair together in a pattern. Second step the hair is back-combed, producing a tight-nit foundation for growing locks. The third step involves palm-rolling the lock. Especially beneficial with hair that is resistant to locking.

[32] Dreadlocks are prohibited by the military. Know the policies and be aware of the laws and your rights!

Building A Free-Form Foundation

Personality:
- Patient personality
- Strong, confident personality
- Trail blazer
- Independent thinker
- Trend setter
- Artsy personality
- Eclectic
- Holistic ideals
- Extremely Patient
- May prefer self-maintenance

Hair Texture:
- Type 4
- All hair types, once foundation is locked

Advantage:
- Extreme shrinkage, frizz and lack of control of hair
- For a thin haired locker, this style will swell and frizz quickly, giving a full appearance
- No foundation pattern to worry about
- Can easily be self-maintained with at least ¼ inch of hair and longer
- No time to install, just wash and go

Disadvantage:
- Extreme shrinkage, frizz and lack of control of hair
- Only Type 4 textures can free-form from installation successfully (without any intervention)
- Societal perceptions as hair transforms into locks
- Lock sizes are variable and inconsistent
- Hair frequently unravels until locked
- Military does not permit dreadlocks[33]

Types of Free-form locks[1]:
Organic
Free-form
Semi-free form

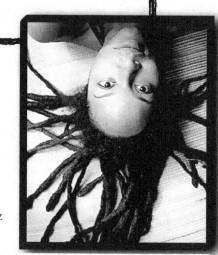

FREE-FORM OR ORGANIC LOCKS

Freeform ($0.00)

[33]Dreadlocks are prohibited by the military. Know the policies and be aware of the laws and your rights!

Building A Braidlock Foundation

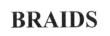

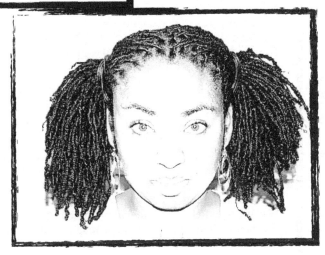

Braids
$$

Personality:

•Comfortable with braids
•Patient personality
•May have concerns about lock appearance
•Wants to minimize the side effects of the locking process
•Prefers to control frizz and expansion as lock morphs from braids to locks
•Wants the versatility of loose hair
•May want Sisterlocks™ or Brotherlocks™ but limited on funds
•May prefer self-maintenance

Hair Texture:

•Type 3, 4
•Type 1, 2, 3, braids may be step one in 3-step combination method

Advantage:

•Tension can be adjusted to address varying degrees of textures
•Most employment and military policies allow for braids
- Size of locks can be controlled
- Lock transformation is minimized, often avoiding detection
- Process may avoid detection if policies are in place to prohibit dreadlocks
- Can be used in 3-step combination method, as the first step, with back-combing as the second step
- Hair should not unravel
- Can easily be self-maintained with one to two inches of hair and longer

Disadvantage:

- Pattern remains for a longer amount of time than any other installation foundation. Pattern disappears anywhere from month eight to year four. However, the new growth minimizes the braid pattern as the braid condenses to half of an inch to an inch at maturity, at the end of the lock.
- Military does not permit dreadlocks[34].
- End of the lock may grow wider than the new growth, if maintained by interlocking/latching, over time
- Installation time depends on length and partings[35]

Type of Braids:

3-Strand
Underhand
Overhand
French
Herringbone
Box
Bread

---

[34]Dreadlocks are prohibited by the military. Know the policies and be aware of the laws and your rights!

[35]Six inches of hair will take approximately ten hours to complete.

Building A Coil Foundation

COILS

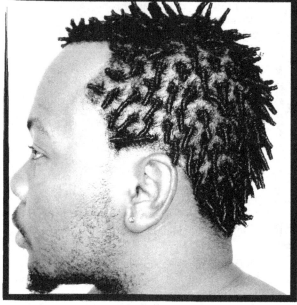

Coils
$

Personality Profile:
- Traditional locker wanting a traditional experience
- Extremely patient personality
- Open to stylist assistance
- Relaxed personality, flexible and confident
- May want to care for own hair

Hair Texture: Type 4

Advantage:
- Traditional locks
- Transforms to locks quickly, no pattern issues
- Coils form into cylindrical locks easily
- Can easily be self-maintained
- Relatively quick to install, 5 min-1.5 hour
- ¼ inch of hair is the minimum requirement to begin with certain rubbing methods

Disadvantage:
- Difficult to wash and style hair first 0-3 months post installation
- Unravels if wet
- Must be comfortable with side effect of frizzy hair
- Military does not permit dreadlocks[36]
- Size of locks may vary
- Societal perceptions as hair transforms into locks
- Hair should be two inches or shorter. Anything longer will not lock well.

Type of Coil:
- Brush
- Washcloth
- Applicator-applied
- Rat-tail Comb
- Fingers
- Nubian locks/China bumps

---

[36]Dreadlocks are prohibited by the military. Know the policies and be aware of the laws and your rights!

LATCHED/ INTERLOCKED

Building An Interlocked Foundation

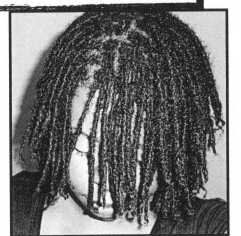

Interlock ($$$$)

Personality:
- May have concerns about lock appearance
- Wants to minimize the side effects of the locking process
- Prefers to control frizz and expansion as locks transform
- Wants versatility of loose hair, without tangling challenges
- Likes the look of Sisterlocks™/Brotherlocks™ without the investment
- Likes the look of manicured locks
- Aware of installation cost and willing to pay
- Low degree of interest in self- maintenance, but may be there if locker has a high skill base of the interlocking process.

Texture:
- Type 3, 4
- Type 1, 2, some 3s textures may be step two in a 3-step combination method for tightening.

Advantage:
- Tension can be adjusted to address varying degrees of textures.
- Can be used in 3-step combination method, as the first step, with backcombing as the second step, rolling as the third step.
- Inconspicuous pattern is not a problem, lock forms quickly.
- Hair resists unraveling
- Can be installed on hair an inch long hair and longer.

Disadvantage:
- Military does not permit dreadlocks[37]
- Must know the technique and be coordinated and systematic with the technique or have locks maintained by stylist
- Locks will go through traditional lock changes
- Installation time of twelve to twenty hours
- Societal perceptions

Type:
- Crochet hook
- Crochet needle
- Hair bead tool
- 2.5 inch hair pin
- Nappylock Tool™
- Hands

---

[37]Dreadlocks are prohibited by the military. Know the policies and be aware of the laws and your rights!

Building A Backcomb Lock Foundation

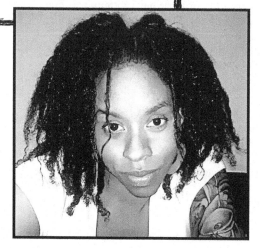

BACKCOMBED

Backcomb*($$ will depend on technique)

Personality:
- Daring
- Willing to take risks
- Artsy
- Relaxed personality, confident, not concerned about appearance
- Strong, confident personality
- Trail blazer
- Trend setter
- If hair is highly textured, tightly coiled (Type 4), no interest in stylist
- If hair is straight or wavy (Type 1, 2, 3) usually interested in stylist assistance

Hair Texture:
- Type 3, 4

Advantage:
- Instant locks!
- No pattern, lock formation easily forms
- Hair should not unravel
- Can be used as step two in 3-step combination process to lock in straight, wavy texture
- Length of hair two to four inches or longer to install
- Installation time of two to four hours or less, depends on size and partings

Disadvantage:
- Military does not permit dreadlocks[38]
- Aesthetics may be challenged by employee policies
- Varying sized of locks
- Societal perceptions
- Locks are not uniform

Types:
- Small-tooth comb
- Rat-tailed comb
- Finger coils

---

[38]Dreadlocks are prohibited by the military. Know the policies and be aware of the laws and your rights!

Building A Sisterlock™ Foundation

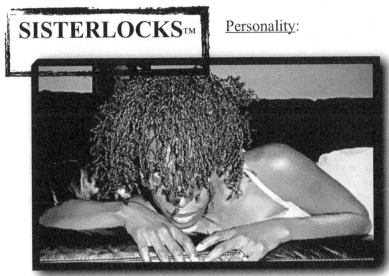

SISTERLOCKS™

Sisterlocks™ Brotherlocks™
($$$$$)

<u>Personality</u>:

- Self-confident, independent, self-loving
- May be an older women ready to embrace self[39].
- May have concerns about appearance
- Wants to minimize the side effects of the locking process
- Prefers to control frizz and expansion as lock transforms to maturity
- Prefers maintenance by a certified consultant
- Wants the versatility of loose hair
- Transitioner with permed hair, not ready to give up length of hair to go natural

<u>Texture</u>:
- Type 3, 4

<u>Advantage</u>:
- Tension can be adjusted to address varying degrees of textures
- Pattern is not an issue with lock appearance
- Lock morphogenesis is minimized and goes through a different, less noticeable process
- Versatility of loose hair
- At least 1.5 inches (or longer) of chemical free hair needed to installs
- Long locks said not to cause excessive weight
- Consultants specifically trained to start locks on chemically processed hair as well as chemical-free virgin hair[40]
- Strong network of Sisterlockers™ world wide

<u>Disadvantage</u>:
- Cost! Installation is determined upon length of hair and tightenings every four to six weeks.
- Maintained only with Sisterlock™ tool and performed by certified consultant to continue to be called Sisterlocks™.
- Some complain of extreme thinning, breaking from fragile locks.
- Must stop using oily products.
- Hair is extremely susceptible to damage if not properly cared for with the Sisterlocks™ product line.
- Military known to deny these locks, categorizing them as dreadlocks[41].
- Controversy with traditional lockers due to cost, regimen and maintenance requirements.
- Certified consultants are difficult to find.
- Installation time of twelve to twenty hours.

<u>Types</u>:
- Sisterlocks™ small/medium/large
- Brotherlocks™ (large Sisterlocks™)

---

[39]Cornwell, Joanne. That Hair Thing. 2nd Edition ed. San Diego: Sisterlocks. Pub, 2009. Print.

[40]All locks can be started with chemically processed hair; however the strength of the hair at the line of demarcation may be compromised and this may lead to a weaker foundation upon lock maturity. The exception is Sisterlocks™.

[41]Dreadlocks are prohibited by the military. Know the policies and be aware of the laws and your rights!

Once the lock foundation is installed, the locker has four to six weeks to decide what method to use to tighten the new growth. New growth is hair that emerges from the scalp and best recognized as the loose hair growing under the locks. Hair grows half of an inch every month, about seven to eight inches a year depending upon hair health by free-forming, twisting/palm-rolling or interlocking. If hair is Type 4, the new growth will lock independently of the manipulation, impacting the shape of the lock. Just as there are choices when installing locks, there are choices to maintain the locks. When hair is successfully tightened, the scalp is visible. Four weeks is the minimum between tightenings; however, the locker can go longer, but no more than eight weeks unless free-forming. Lock installation selection and new growth maintenance are equally vital to affect the shape of the mature lock. Keep in mind the preceding personality profiles may or may not be characteristic of the locker's personality. Locking is an individual art form and dependent upon many factors[42]. In addition, as with the Combination-Installation Personality Chart (Fig. 3.2), one's view of what is messy to one and acceptable to another will vary, based upon personal preference. What may look unkempt and messy to one, may be another's preference. Use this resource as a guide. Apply judgment and knowledge of the locker to formulate the final decision. Fortunately, most traditional installations and tightening techniques are not absolute and can be changed. The only exception is Sisterlocks™ or Brotherlocks™. In this case, installation is performed by a certified consultant. However, many have chosen to maintain on their own, switching the technique to interlocking, using a different tool, combining, even twisting; however, may not be considered Sisterlocks™ when manipulated outside of Sisterlock™ guidelines.

---

[42]The suggestions presented in this manual do not negate individual choice, they are a tool to use as a guide.

Commitment

Webster defines commitment as keeping a promise. Reliable. Dedicated. Unchanging.

I define commitment as the ability to be true to a purpose, cause, self and others.

Your locks will tell you whether they want to seal or curl or just be.
Shhh, listen and learn who they are and appreciate them for the beauty they bring.

They grow because you trust. They grow because you listen. As they grow, you learn. when you learn, share, so others can grow.

Become one with the texture. A cottony-wool blend of the best quality hair on the planet. Strong, yet sensitive. Durable, yet, fragile.

There really are locks on the other side of the buds, frizz and mess and they are beautiful!

Locking the hair is a commitment to self. And, you are worth it.

mgeorge©2010

PART TWO

HOW TO

CREATE BEAUTIFUL LOCKS

4

Setting The Grid
&
Building From The Roots
The Parts

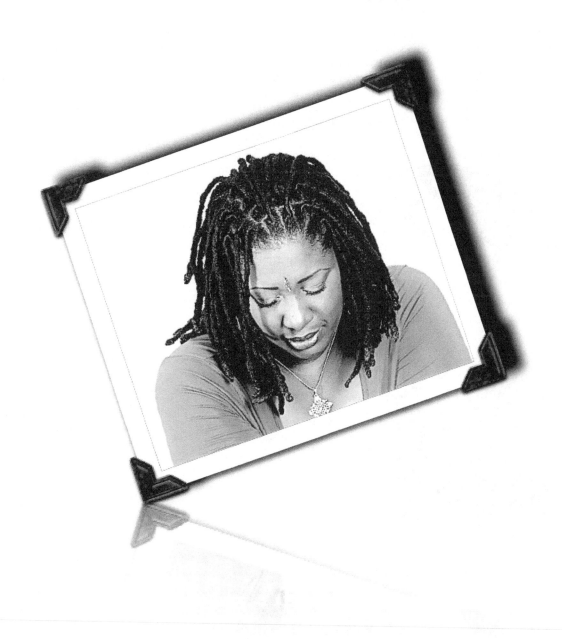

THE GRID

After choosing the lock foundation, the lock sections can be parted into various formations: diamonds, brick laid, squares, pyramids or circles before installation. In the beginning, fancy parts will look nice; however, all locks, except trademarked Sisterlocks™ can shift and lose their original sectioning. Sisterlocks™ are uniquely installed so the part grid is always uniform unless intentionally changed or if new growth sprouts from a previously stagnant follicle[43]. For any lock, it's important to stay focused on the process and not the parts, because locking becomes a transient process. Choosing a parting for traditional locks is for aesthetic purposes; however, the maintenance technique and the installation foundation synergistically guide the shape of the developing lock.

How to determine the parting size:

After deciding the grid, the pattern of the parting placement, the next step is to decide the parting size. The parting size will form the base of the lock. The base of the lock is the foundation, which the mature lock will develop from. Because it is the root-base of the lock, just like a building, the foundation must be strong to stabilize and maintain the weight of the lock. One half of an inch of new growth emerges from the follicles along the scalp monthly. Each month, or every four to six weeks, the new growth will need to be integrated into the lock, or left to freeform. If the base is smaller than the lock, the root-base will become stressed. Stressed hair breaks. The following guideline will form a strong root-base for traditional lock installation to grow:

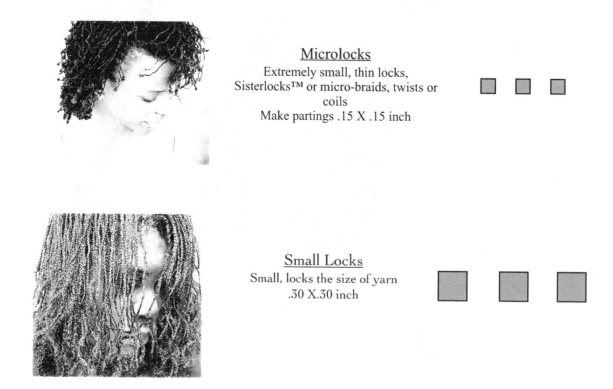

Microlocks
Extremely small, thin locks,
Sisterlocks™ or micro-braids, twists or coils
Make partings .15 X .15 inch

Small Locks
Small, locks the size of yarn
.30 X.30 inch

---

[43]Parts only installed by a certified Sisterlock™ consultant.

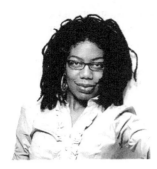

Medium Locks
Pencil size/ straw sized locks
.40 X .40 inch

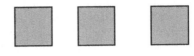

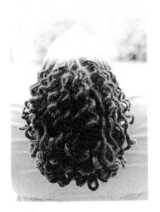

Large Locks
Thick- sized locks
size of a large magic marker
.5 X .5 inch partings or greater

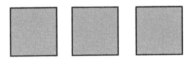

Because partings are an individual preference, it's important to remain flexible with the parting size, because the weight of the lock can grow to the point where the root-base becomes weak. If the root-base becomes weak, it will feel thin and fragile, while holding onto the installation lock by a thread of its former glory. To strengthen the root-bed, adjacent locks need to be combined to form a stronger foundation. Traditional microlocks are an example of a changing root-bed. Traditional microlocks, can begin as small, then enlarged by combining over time. The need to combine will usually occur by month six, when most locks will begin to bud and expand, causing the weight of the lock to exceed the width of the base. The root-base will need to be combined with an adjacent lock's root-base for strength and stability anytime the width of the lock increases past the width of the base of the lock. This technique is called start slow and grow. Aesthetically, the advantage of this technique is the locks will grow, expand and change. This may be an option for lockers that are concerned about getting bored with the same look. It's also easier to combine locks than it is to split locks. Starting slow and growing allows the locker the flexibility to enlarge the locks and change the lock, adding adjacent locks throughout the transformation process.

Because the scalp is dynamic, partings usually change as the living tissue in the scalp changes over time with collagen, fat deposits, aging, hair growth, and the regeneration of new growth. When new hair grows, locks may experience shifting and movement as the scalp transforms with new growth, displacing hair follicles. Follicles are terminal and the number at birth, around 100K is static, it never increases or decreases; however, the hair follicle can die and never produce hair again. When locking, follicles that previously stopped growing hair, often experience regeneration of hair growth from the papilla in the follicle as previously dead follicles rejuvenate with rest and proper nutrition. Always handle highly textured hair with great care!

Knotty Note

Parting Tools:

Manicured hands
Spray bottle with purified water!!
Coated pony tail holders
Duck-billed clips
Scrunchie
Rounded, wide-set comb

Set the Grid

1. Spritz the hair with purified water or a softening agent, such as Aloe Vera juice to soften the hair cuticles. Apply and massaged into the scalp before handling the hair.

2. Separate and secure the hair into 4 X 4 inch working sections with a wide toothed comb with rounded tips. Gather and secure the hair with gentle hair utensils: covered ponytail holders, duck billed clips or a secure braid.

3. Make the part at the nape (back) of the head and begin laying the foundation. Secure the installed foundation away from the loose hair and proceed.

The grid can be laid out in different formations. Make a note of the formation chosen in the lock chart:

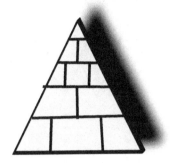

Fig. 4.1 <u>Bricklay</u>- Setting parts with triangular shapes radiating from the crown.

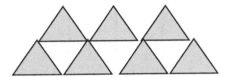

Fig. 4.2 <u>Triangle</u>-Alternate partings in a triangular formation.

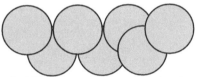

Fig. 4.3 <u>Circle</u>-Partings are arranged in circular formations.

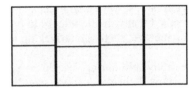

Fig. 4.4 <u>Squares</u>-Partings are arranged in squares.

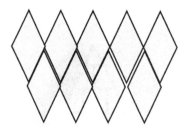

Fig.4.5 <u>Diamonds</u>-Partings are arranged in diamonds.

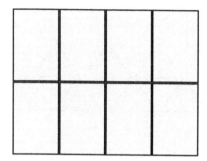

Fig 4.6 <u>Rectangles</u>-Partings are arranged in rectangles.

The size of the root-base is important to the size of the emerging lock. Will the size of the root-base solely determine the size of the mature lock? No. The size of the mature lock is dependent upon: density of the hair and scalp, texture and the tightening technique chosen. There are many lockers with inch-sized parting root-base sections, with a small lock shaft. Conversely, locks can have a large root-base with a large lock shaft. The best way to guide the shape of the maturing lock is to choose a tightening method that will allow locks to expand-such as palm-rolling or a method that pacts the lock into a tight matrix, reducing the size, such as interlocking in a four point or six point rotation.

If the maturing lock is too large, locks can be safely split during year three. Year three is important because it usually takes thirty-six months for locks to begin to show their true, mature size. Splitting is a long, tedious process. The advantage is that the locker does not need to start over. Splitting is only done on interlocked locks. Combining is the process of joining two adjacent lock root-bases[44]. Combining or splitting will also change the original grid formation. The beauty of the journey is witnessing who the locks will become with guidance and time.

---

[44]See The Lock Challenge Chapter for instructions on splitting and combining locks.

5

The Root of The Matter
Lock Installation and Maintenance

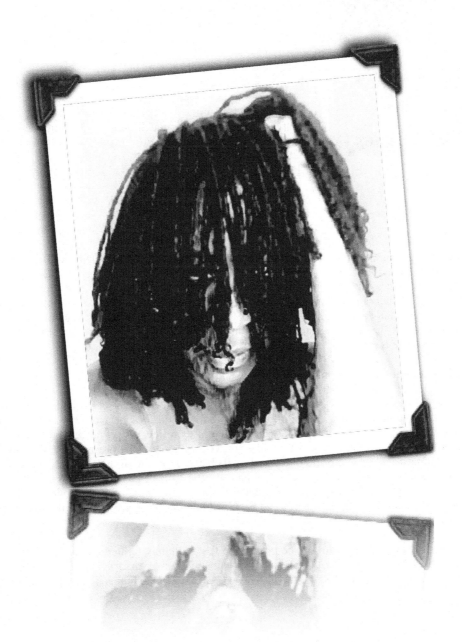

Tending The Root-Bed

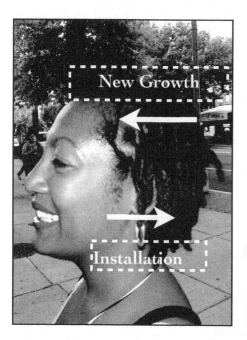

After the locks are installed, all the right questions are asked, four to six weeks later new growth will emerge from the scalp. Then, it's time to decide what to do with that new growth! The new growth is important, because it is the new growth that will become the future lock. As the new growth emerges, the foundational section will condense, shrink and lose its pattern, forming a lock 'anchor' that becomes the platform network of woven hair, crucial to the inner-matrix of the locked core. This lock anchor will send signals establishing the foundation of the lock. When installed, the foundation of an emerging lock (braids, coils, two strand etc...) is just a hairstyle for about one to two months. On average after two months, hair will begin to lock; and, this simple foundation will dictate the direction of the future lock and the maintenance or tightening technique will mold the shape of the future lock.

Maintenance options come in three basic forms: palm-rolling, interlocking or free-forming and will directly impact whether the locks appear manicured, groomed, or fuzzy, loose and freely-formed. Locking is exciting, and a long-term process; therefore, it's important to choose a foundation and tightening method compatible to the locker's biological traits of the hair, as well as lifestyle. Determining the skills, methods and costs associated with lock maintenance is covered in detail in this section.

When it comes to tightening the new growth, it will depend on the aesthetic preference of the locker. How does the locker want to appear to the world? How does the locker want to appear to self? Is remaining neat and manicured important? Does the locker prefer to free-form or semi-free form the new growth? Is the locker an avid sportsman, needing frequent washings? Does the locker have the skills and capabilities to self-maintain the new growth? Does the locker prefer to have a stylist maintain or self-maintain? How will the locker's lifestyle impact lock presentation? These are all unique, individual decisions, just like lock installation is a uniquely individual choice. One technique does not fit all; however, unlike installation, the tightening method can be changed throughout the life of the locks. This process and transformation is dynamic. Another consideration is cost. Lock maintenance costs can vary widely from 0$ with free-formed locks to $50/hr tightening sessions with some Sisterlocks™ consultants.

Be aware that there are differences between the new growth and locked hair. New growth is hair that is loose and not locked. If left alone, the new growth will eventually lock, when hair is highly textured. In most cases, the new growth will be cultivated into a pattern by twisting, free-forming or interlocking to set the lock, as mentioned in *The Now What? Chapter*. As the new growth comes in, the length will begin to appear cm by cm, inch by inch. The former foundation will continue to shorten, condense into a stub of its former glory; however, the new growth must enter the process of locking and integrate into the older locked inner-matrix before transforming into locks. The original shrinkage continues and the end or tip of the lock will change. The end of the lock/tip may remain open and coiled and never seal, depending upon the texture of the hair. If little balls of hair form at the end of the lock, leave them alone. That is shed hair. Most hair-balls will form a sealed lock tip, many will shed away when shampooing. The hair is busy sprouting and budding (releasing shed hair) and locking for approximately the first year and a half (covered in The Lock Evolution Chapter).

There are a few consistent rules to apply to root-bed care. The first is to only tighten the loose, root-bed, every four to six weeks. Do not challenge this rule. Tightening the hair any sooner than every four to six weeks would compromise the health of the hair. Just like a chemical relaxer breaks down the bonds in hair, leaving hair inherently weak and prone to damage, overly maintaining the root-bed will do the same thing. This will cause the hair to weaken on a microscopic level, tear, and eventually break off. Locks can be lost from over manipulating, so don't be a twisted sister, or brother. Give the hair the time it needs to rest, then tighten in the fourth to sixth week post the last maintenance period. A weak lock shaft leads to weak locks, period.

The first year, it is important to keep a four to six week tightening regimen, unless free-forming organic locks. Waiting longer than four to six weeks to tighten can compromise and weaken the root-bed, as hair begins to crawl (loose hair in the root-bed spreading to other root-beds) into adjacent root-beds. Another way to keep the root-bed strong and healthy is to spritz daily with a hair growth preparation, followed by massages. Hair should only be tightened on damp hair, preferably after washing the hair. If the hair is dry or dries during the tightening session, continue to keep damp with the hair growth preparation spritz. A healthy root-bed equals happy follicles and happy follicles equal new hair growth! Finally, only hydrophilic, water-soluble, ingredients should be used on locks. This chapter will instruct the locker 'how' to perform the specific tightening methods based upon lifestyle and preference.

Knotty Note

Main Rules for Tightening the Hair

1. Wait a minimum of 4-6 weeks between tightenings.
2. Only use hydrophilic hair preparations during tightening.
3. Only tighten damp hair.
4. Spritz with a hair preparation to keep roots damp throughout the latching process.
5. Never tighten through the same hole twice.

Step 1: Prepare the new growth/root-bed (for all techniques)

1. Spritz the hair lightly, making it easier to work on the new growth.

2. Examine the new growth and determine if the root-bed of adjacent locks need to be separated. If the root-beds are sticking, they may need to be gently popped and separated. Pop/pull apart any hair that may have moved from its parting section to another parting section. When hair creeps (also known as crawling or become married) to another section, parts are still visible; but, some hairs have strayed across the part line and seem to 'stick' to another root-bed section[45]. To separate locks, spritz the root-bed, then gently tug the locks apart until the hair has separated from the adjoining section. Continue with the process. If some hairs seem to creep to adjoining locks, the root-beds will not separate. The last resort is to snip the stray hair with a pair of scissors, separating the root beds, restoring the parting sections.

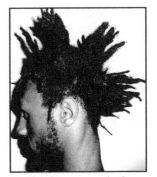

Jordan is an organic free-former of the truest form. His prefers the roots to stick and mat.

The second scenario is a matted root-bed. When the new growth is matted, the partings are not seen and the root-beds are joined. All of the adjacent locks appear merged as one. The new growth appears to be a uniform Afro, with no distinct difference between one lock's root-bed to another. This results in slippage that has grown either faster than normal, or the locker has forsaken the necessary four to

---

[45]See The Lock Challenge Chapter.

six week tightening session. Matting is a result of hairs that creep over forming a network of meshed hair. To separate matted root-beds, place a drop of the lock preparation gel[46] on the fingertips of the index finger and thumb and massage into the loose, new growth, spritz and gently tug until the root-beds are separated from one another. Secure one lock from another by putting the hair into four quadrants, secured with coated ponytail holders or duck billed clips. This will take some time. It's important to always be gentle and patient. When separating adjacent locks, the sound of separating the root-bed sounds like paper ripping. Be gentle and try not to actually rip the hair. It's safe as long as the root-bed is dampened with the spritz or water. When separating, look carefully and make sure the hair is not tearing. It's a skill that must be learned with careful observance, practice and listening. To resolve matting that won't separate, clip the joined hairs with scissors or combine them at the root-bed[47]. Combining locks is the process of combining the root-bed of adjacent locks. Combining also fortifies locks that have grown heavier than the supporting root-bed. Combining can also be done to increase the size of the lock. Combining is a positive technique that contributes to healthy locks. Snipping the creeping hairs is not. Snipping, cutting stray hairs, can weaken the root-bed, compromising the health of the lock. To avoid snipping, another four to six week growth cycle followed with popping, may separate the root-bed. If not, snip as the method of last resort. Make a note of the root-bed, the techniques and the preparations used to strengthen the root-bed in the lock chart. Advise the locker to avoid matting and creeping with regular tightenings every four to six weeks.

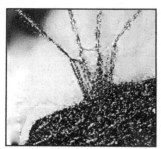

Ouch! The roots are matted and creeping to other root-beds. This will hurt when popping!

B. Step 2: Examine the direction of the locks (for all techniques)[48]

Regardless of the tightening positions used, assess the direction of the lock formation, by the Directional, Weathervane or Clock Method. All directions can uniformly be assessed from back to front of the head. The most common ways to reference locks are by the following three methods. Most methods interchangeably use the same nomenclature, choose one that works the best:

Directional/Weathervane Method
Locks are tightened using the weathervane positions: North/South/East/West; positional directions: right/left/top/down and body positions: shoulders, top of head, ears to guide the rotation.

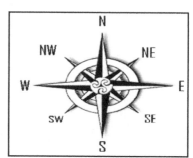

Fig. 5.1 A weathervane used for determining lock direction.

Stationary anatomical features allow the rotations to have a consistent point of reference to anchor and guide the lock through the latching process. The only difference in the methods is what the positions are called. Make note of the method used in the lock chart for future reference. If latching with fingers, just push the end of the lock through the proper entry position and pull through with fingers, following the same directions. Latching with fingers will secure the new growth, eliminate unraveling and give a less manicured look, blending the new growth easily into the installed lock. Typically, more new growth will be needed to complete a full finger latch

---

[46]See The Holistic Hair Care Chapter.

[47]See The Lock Challenge Chapter for directions.

[48]Many lockers practice the art of locking in various directions. There is no wrong or right way to interlock locks. The key is consistency, proper tension, and proper maintenance. For the sake of simplicity, only two methods and their respective directions will be addressed, please see Fig. 5.3, 5.4, 5.5 for pictorial explanation, and later in this chapter for full directions.

rotation. If the hair unravels, bunching and slipping can occur, especially if the texture is straight and wavy in the Type 1 to Type 3 range. Bunching and slipping can occur from the use of conditioning products during the early stages of locking as well. Using herbal teas for conditioning can help to counter this side effect caused by common hair oils and conditioners or texture. Reversing the rotation in a counter-clockwise direction can also help to counter this occurrence. Assess each area for texture variances along the scalp and set the rotations accordingly, to maximize lock integrity.

Clock Method:

Locks are tightened in a counterclockwise or clockwise direction. The clockwise direction continues in the direction of the hands of a clock in a 12/3/6/9 direction. The counterclockwise direction is the opposite and continues in the direction of the hands of a clock in a 12/9/6/3 direction. In conjunction, body positions are used to guide the rotations; however, the rotations are called according to the time points on a clock.

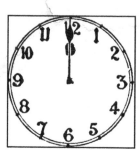

Fig. 5.2 Clocks can help guide the direction of the latch

Once the direction of the locks has been determined, make a note of it in the lock chart. This is one of the most important steps! If palm-rolled locks are rolled counter to the original direction, they can unravel, at worst, or the action can disturb the locking process. If latched locks are latched in the wrong direction, the locking process can be disturbed as well. The new growth won't unravel; however, the wrong direction will set the hair back in terms of length. Being consistent with the direction of the retightening of the new growth is very important and it should be noted.

Quadrant Positioning

Posterior Quadrant:

The posterior plane is at the back of the head. When retightening the hair, it's best to pick a quadrant to always begin with. When beginning the latch at the back of the head, the first rotation is from the West entry point position, this position is from the left ear, exiting East, towards the right ear (Fig. 5.5). The locks will lie down *towards the back* of the head when the last rotation is completed at the fourth position point.

Right Front Sagittal Quadrant:

The frontal plane, front of the head, is split into two quadrants, the right side and the left side of the body(saggital means right and left side of the body). When beginning the latch at the front right quadrant, the first rotation is from the West entry point position. This position is from the back of the head, exiting East, towards the forehead. The locks will lie down *towards the right ear* when the full rotation is complete (Fig. 5.3).

Left Front Sagittal Quadrant:

The frontal plane, front of head) is split into two quadrants, the right side and the left side of the body (saggital means right and left side of the body). When beginning the latch at the front left quadrant, the first rotation is from the West entry point position. This position is from the forehead, exiting East, towards the back of the head. The locks will lay down *towards the left ear* when the full rotation is complete (Fig. 5.4).

Unlike *The Now What? Chapter*, this chapter looks at the specific lock installation considerations and maintenance. The following profiles will help the locker to specifically decide the preferred installation and tightening technique, and tailor it for personality, lifestyle, preference, skill set, and hair texture.

CREATING BEAUTIFUL LOCKS ON A DIME!

Locking The Foundation

by
Interlocking/ Tool-Latching/ Crocheting/Sewing/Finger Latching

($$$$)

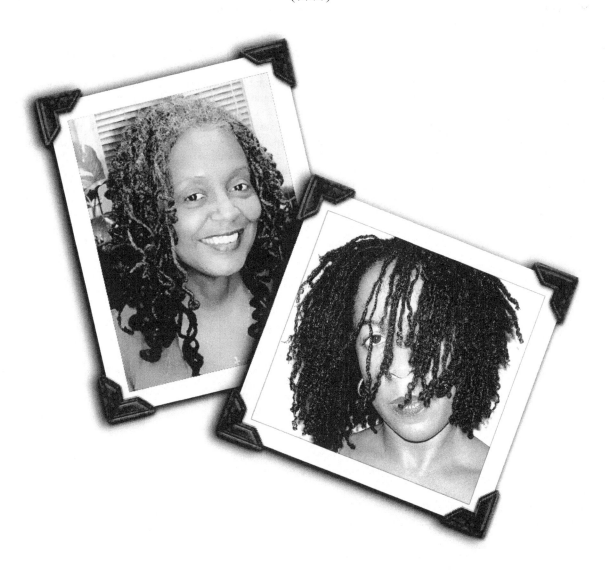

Interlocking the new growth requires a high skill set level and a confidence with the interlocking process, also known as latching, crocheting, sewing, finger-latching. The advantage of interlocking is that it secures the hair, there's no product build up, and the root-bed will not unravel. When latching, make sure there is enough new growth for a full rotation. The pattern of interlocked locks will remain stationary as long as the direction of the rotation is not changed. If the pattern changes, it can result in a difference in the lock appearance. It may not manifest to the naked eye, because the network of intertwined hair is very forgiving. What is noticeable is a change in length, as the curl pattern readjusts. When measured, the length may be noticeably shorter. In addition, a change in the number of entry points for a latch rotation or alternating between twisting and latching can result in physical differences. The former will result in locks with a small circumference. The latter, will result in alternating swelling and thin spots along the lock. Both actions could result in non-uniform locks and stressed areas. The tool can change without consequence to the lock formation. In other words, switching between tools has not been *proven* to change the appearance of a lock.

A full rotation is latching with four entry points. A half rotation is latching with two entry points. When locks are maintained by a stylist, the stylists will usually determine the price based upon the number of rotations to complete tightening the loose, newly, grown roots. To keep the price reasonable, keep up with tightenings every four to six weeks! One full rotation usually takes four to six weeks to grow and equates roughly half of an inch of new growth. Because hair grows at different rates, a full rotation may not exist uniformly across the scalp. If this is the case, make a note of the growth variations in the lock chart. It is the discretion of the stylist and locker whether to proceed with a half rotation or a full rotation. When beginning each tightening session, stay consistent and always begin the rotation at the same entry point, regardless of where the last session ended. To begin latching, spritz the root-bed often, tighten the locks section by section, use clips to isolate the working lock from the other root-beds, secure hairs that creep and crawl over from other root-beds. Once the entire head is complete, repeat in four to six weeks and continue the pattern. Begin latching at the same quadrant on the head each time to reduce creeping and crawling. Integrate loose hairs into the latched lock with a tool or hand[49].

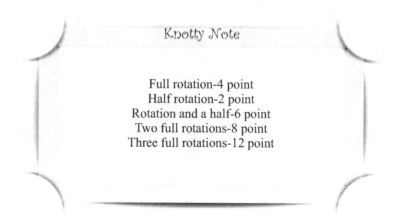

Knotty Note

Full rotation-4 point
Half rotation-2 point
Rotation and a half-6 point
Two full rotations-8 point
Three full rotations-12 point

---

[49]See section at the end of chapter on how to integrate loose hairs into the lock.

Personality[50]:

- Manicured maintenance is important (unless finger-locked, convenience is preference)
- May exhibit a controlling personality
- Impatient, detail oriented
- Wants locks with minimal drama

Who?

- Corporate employee concerned about appearance
- College student with active lifestyle
- Mom with busy lifestyle
- Gentleman with active sports life
- Helmet jobs
- Military service employee
- Sports/active lifestyle
- Swimmer

Textures:

- All textures
- Higher tolerance to pain

Skill Set:

- Highly skilled with tool use and methodology
- If finger latched, loose lock, minimal skill

Result:

- Traditionally seen with small locks, with a small diameter. Rotations can be manipulated to produce larger locks. Neat appearance but not a distinct look like twisting/palm-rolling or 2-step twist combination method.

Advantage:

- No product required
- Locks do not unravel

Disadvantage:

- Stray hairs not integrated into lock[51]
- Not defined when tightened
- Installation time depends on size of locks and partings, two to five hours average.
- High skill set required

Supplies:

- Manicured hands
- Duck-billed clips, coated ponytail holders
- Spray bottle of healthy hair spritz
- Towel
- Manicured fingers (prevents snagging)

 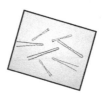 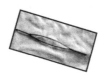

---

[50]General observations

[51]Two-step twist combination method can prevent stray hairs.

Do it! Interlocking *via* the Directional Method

1st Rotation from the Back, Posterior Plane (Fig. 5.5)
Enter West/ exit East / loop or thread the lock/ pull out /West

Enter from the West entry point closest to the left ear, the tip of the tool enters the loose new growth on the left side of the head. The left ear is the reference point. Push the tool through the new growth from left towards the right ear. Then, pull the tool down until it stops at the beginning of the lock at the new growth line of demarcation. The line of demarcation for locks is the point where the new growth meets the lock. This is the starting point to begin the rotation. Before exiting on the East side of the head, towards the right ear, thread the end of the lock through the tool:

- If the tool is a 2.5 inch hair pin it will be pushed through the U-shaped tip.
- If the tool is a crochet needle, make sure the hook *and* the latch is all the way on the other side, the hair will be secured inside of the hook and the door of the latch pushed shut, then pull through.
- If the tool is the shape of a threading needle, the end of the lock will be pushed through the hole.

Once the end of the lock is secured inside of the latch tool, pull the end of the hair back out, towards the West position which is towards the left ear. If the locks are long enough (longer than four inches) continue the latching rotation, leaving the end of the lock threaded inside of the latch tool hole[52]. If the locks are short, take the end of the lock out of the latch tool and continue with the latching rotation, by rethreading each time.

2nd Rotation (Fig. 5.5)
Enter North exit South/ loop or thread the lock/pull out North

Enter from the top of the head, North position, the tip of the tool enters the loose new growth on the top side of the head. The top of the head is the reference point. Push the tool through the new growth from top of the head towards the shoulders. Then, pull the tool down until it stops at the beginning of the lock at the new growth line of demarcation. The line of demarcation for locks is the point where the new growth meets the lock. This is the starting point to begin the rotation. Before exiting from the shoulders, thread the end of the lock through the tool:

- If the tool is a 2.5 inch hair pin it will be pushed through the U-shaped tip.
- If the tool is a crochet needle, make sure the hook *and* the latch is all the way on the other side, the hair will be secured inside of the hook and the door of the latch pushed shut, then pull through.
- If the tool is the shape of a threading needle, the end of the lock will be pushed through the hole.

Once the end of the lock is secured inside of the latch tool, pull the end of the hair back out towards the top of the head. If the locks are long enough, (longer than four inches) continue the latching rotation, leaving the end of the lock threaded inside of the latch tool hole[53]. If the locks are short, take the end of the lock out of the latch tool and continue with the latching rotation, by rethreading each time.

---

[52]If the tool is a crochet needle, the end of the lock will need to be threaded at each loop point. If it's a tool with a hole, continue the threading rotation continuously.

[53]If the tool is a crochet needle, the end of the lock will need to be threaded at each loop point. If it's a tool with a hole, continue the threading rotation continuously.

3rd Rotation (Fig 5.5)
Enter East/ exit West/ loop or thread the lock/ East

Enter from the East side, the tip of the tool enters the loose new growth on the right side of the head. The right ear is the reference point. Push the tool through the new growth from right towards the left ear. Then, pull the tool down until it stops at the beginning of the lock at the new growth line of demarcation. The line of demarcation for locks is the point where the new growth meets the lock. This is the starting point of the rotation. As the tool exits on the East side of the head, towards the right ear, thread the end of the lock through the tool:

- · If the tool is a 2.5 inch hair pin push the end of the lock through the U-shaped tip.
- · If the tool is a crochet needle, make sure the hook *and* the latch is all the way on the other side, the hair will be secured inside of the hook and the door of the latch pushed shut, then pull the end of the lock through.
- · If the tool is a form of latch tool the shape of a threading needle, push the end of the lock through the hole.

Once the end of the lock is secured inside of the latch tool, pull the end of the hair back out towards the right ear. If the locks are long enough, (longer than four inches) continue the latching rotation, leaving the end of the lock threaded inside of the latch tool[54]. If the locks are short, take the end of the lock out of the latch tool and continue with the latching rotation, by rethreading each time.

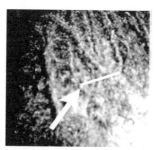

The Line of Demarcation is where the tool will stop and the latch will start here and end at the scalp.

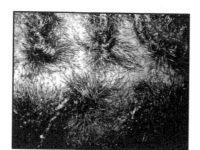

Tightened, latched locks!

4th Rotation (Fig 5.5)
Enter South/ exit North/ loop or thread the lock/ pull out South

Enter from the direction of the shoulder region, the South point along the head, the tip of the tool enters the loose new growth on the lower side of the head. The shoulders are the reference point. Push the tool through the new growth from the bottom towards the top of the head, the North point. Then, pull the tool down until it stops at the beginning of the lock at the new growth line of demarcation. The line of demarcation for locks is the point where the new growth meets the lock. This is the starting point to begin the rotation. Before exiting the top side of the head, thread the end of the lock through the tool:

- · If the tool is a 2.5 inch hair pin push the end of the lock through the U-shaped tip.
- · If the tool is a crochet needle, make sure the hook *and* the latch is all the way on the other side, the hair will be secured inside of the hook and the door of the latch pushed shut, then pull the end of the lock through.

---

[54]If the tool is a crochet needle, the end of the lock will need to be threaded at each loop point. If it's a tool with a hole, continue the threading rotation continuously.

· If the tool is a form of latch tool the shape of a threading needle, push the end of the lock through the hole.

Once the end of the lock is secured inside of the latch tool, pull the end of the hair back out towards the bottom of the head. If the locks are long enough, (longer than four inches) continue the latching rotation, leaving the end of the lock threaded inside of the latch tool[55]. If the locks are short, take the end of the lock out of the latch tool and continue with the latching rotation, by rethreading each time. If the last latch is within an eighth of an inch to the scalp, stop and move on to the next lock.

For the purpose of clarity, the anatomical positions of the head are important and helpful for consistent record keeping (Fig. 5.3, 5.4, 5.5).

_____

[55]If the tool is a crochet needle, the end of the lock will need to be threaded at each loop point. If it's a tool with a hole, continue the threading rotation continuously.

Knotty Note

Summary of Directional Method:[50]

- Enter West/ exit East / loop or thread the lock/ pull out /West
- Enter North exit South/ loop or thread the lock/pull out North
- Enter East/ exit West/ loop or thread the lock/ East
- Enter South/ exit North/ loop or thread the lock/ pull out South

Rotational Latching Points

Right Saggital
Plane

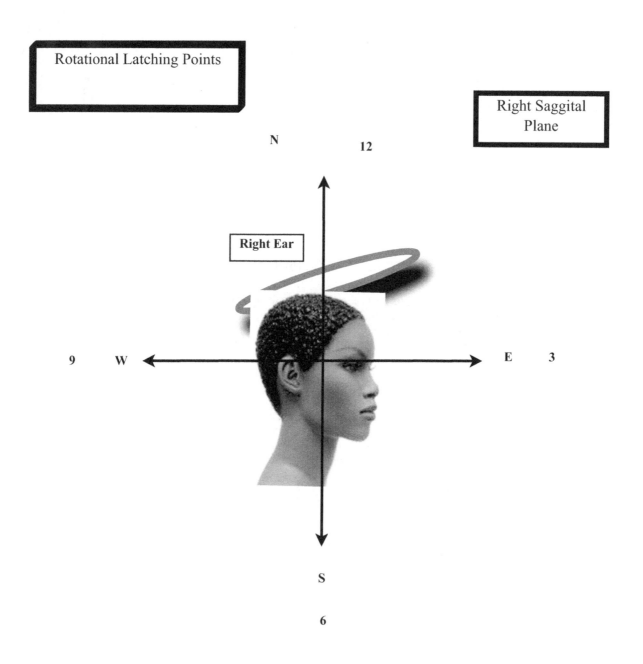

N   12

Right Ear

9   W   E   3

S

6

Fig. 5.3 Planes Split the body into two parts, the right side and left side
of the body.
North-top of head
South-shoulders
East-forehead
West-back of head

Rotational Latching Points

Left Saggital Plane
(left side of body)

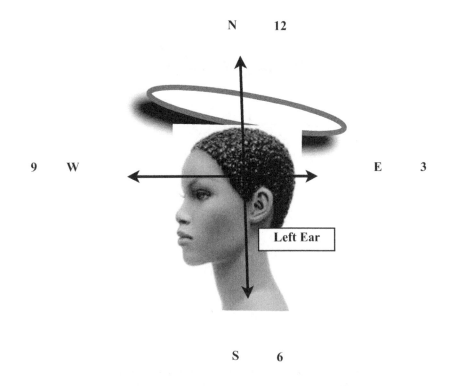

N   12

9   W   E   3

Left Ear

S   6

Fig. 5.4 Planes Split the body into two parts, the right side and left side of the body.
North-Top of head
South-Shoulders
East-Back of head
West-Forehead

CREATING BEAUTIFUL LOCKS ON A DIME!   91

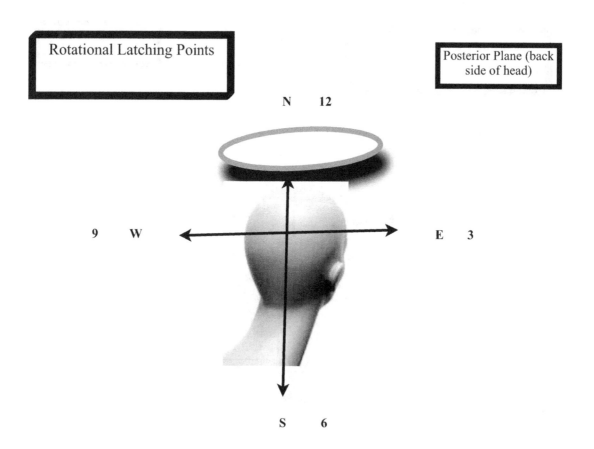

Rotational Latching Points

Posterior Plane (back side of head)

N   12

9   W   E   3

S   6

Fig. 5.5 Planes split the body in two parts, the front of the
body is separated from the back of the body (posterior
position) from the frontal plane (anterior position).
North-Top of head
south-Shoulders
East-Right ear
West-Left ear

Do it! Interlocking via the Clock Method

The clockwise method is the same as the directional method. The only difference is changing the name of the points of entry. There is no difference between the directional and clock methods, just a difference in what the positions are *called*. Make note of the method used in the lock chart for future reference. The clockwise method can effectively be used with highly textured hair in the Type 4 range. The counter-clockwise method is often used with straighter, wavy curl patterns to secure the lock. Assess each area for texture variances along the scalp and set the rotations accordingly to maximize lock integrity, making the latch point rotations begin at 3 o'clock and end at 6 o'clock in a 3/12/9/6 o'clock rotation. If the clock method is continued for a second, third, fourth etc. rotation, continue insertion to the right of each point. The first rotation set would be 9/12/3/6 o'clock rotation. The second rotation set will be 10/1/4/7 o'clock. The third rotation set would be 11/2/5/8 o'clock and so on. Never insert the latch tool through the same hole.

If latching with fingers, just push the end of the lock through the proper entry position and pull through with fingers, following the same directions[56]. Typically, more new growth will be needed to complete a full latch rotation for finger latching. If the hair unravels, bunching and slipping can occur, especially if the texture is a straight or wavy texture in the Type 1 to Type 3 range. Reversing the rotation can help to counter this occurrence by changing a clockwise 9/12/3/6 rotation to a counter-clockwise 6/3/12/9 rotational direction.

For the purpose of clarity, the anatomical positions of the head are important for consistent record keeping (Fig. 5.3, 5.4 and 5.5) for this method as well.

---

[56]If latching with fingers, just push the end of the lock through the proper entry position and pull through with fingers, following the same directions. Typically, more new growth will be needed to complete a full latch rotation for finger latching. If the hair unravels, bunching and slipping can occur, especially if the texture is a looser texture in the Type 1 to Type 3 range. Reversing the rotation can help to counter this occurrence. Assess each area for texture variances along the scalp and set the rotations accordingly to maximize lock integrity.

Do it! Interlocking via the Clock Method[57]

1st Rotation from the back, posterior plane (Fig 5.5)
Enter at 9 o'clock position/ exit and thread or loop the lock at 3 o'clock position/pull out at 9 o'clock position

Enter from the 9 o'clock entry point closest to the left ear, the tip of the tool enters the loose new growth on the left side of the head. The left ear is the reference point. Push the tool through the new growth from left towards the right ear, 3 o'clock. Then, pull the tool down until it stops at the beginning of the lock at the new growth line of demarcation. The line of demarcation for locks is the point where the new growth meets the lock. This is the starting point to begin the rotation. As the tool exits the East side of the head, towards the right ear, thread the end of the lock through the tool:

- If the tool is a 2.5 inch hair pin push the end of the lock through the U-shaped tip.
- If the tool is a crochet needle, make sure the hook *and* the latch is all the way on the other side, the hair will be secured inside of the hook and the door of the latch pushed shut, then pull the end of the lock through.
- If the tool is a form of latch tool the shape of a threading needle, push the end of the lock through the hole.

Once the end of the lock is secured inside of the latch tool, pull the end of the hair back out, towards the 9 o'clock position, which is towards the left ear. If the locks are long enough, (longer than four inches) continue the latching rotation, leaving the end of the lock threaded inside of the latch tool hole[58]. If the locks are short, take the end of the lock out of the latch tool and continue with the latching rotation, by rethreading each time.

2nd Rotation (Fig 5.5)
Enter at 12 o'clock position/ exit and thread or loop the lock at 6 o'clock position/pull out at 12 o'clock position

Enter from the top of the head, 12 o'clock position, the tip of the tool enters the loose new growth on the top side of the head. The top of the head is the reference point. Push the tool through the new growth from 12 o'clock towards 6 o'clock. Then, pull the tool down until it stops at the beginning of the lock at the new growth line of demarcation. The line of demarcation for locks is the point where the new growth meets the lock. This is the starting point to begin the rotation. As the tool exits the bottom side of the head, thread the end of the lock through the tool:

- If the tool is a 2.5 inch hair pin push the end of the lock through the U-shaped tip.
- If the tool is a crochet needle, make sure the hook *and* the latch is all the way on the other side, the hair will be secured inside of the hook and the door of the latch pushed shut, then pull the end of the lock through.
- If the tool is a form of latch tool the shape of a threading needle, push the end of the lock through the hole.

Once the end of the lock is secured inside of the latch tool, pull the end of the hair back out towards the top of the head. If the locks are long enough, (longer than four inches) continue the latching rotation, leaving the end of the

---

[57]Imagine threading a needle with a strand of hair.

[58] If the tool is a crochet needle, the end of the lock will need to be threaded at each loop point. If it's a tool with a hole, continue the threading rotation continuously.

lock threaded inside of the latch tool hole[59]. If the locks are short, take the end of the lock out of the latch tool and continue with the latching rotation, by rethreading each time.

3rd Rotation (Fig 5.5)
Enter at 3 o'clock position/ exit and thread or loop the lock at 9 o'clock position/pull out at 3 o'clock position

Enter from the 3 o'clock position, the tip of the tool enters the loose new growth on the right side of the head at 3 o'clock. The right ear is the reference point. Push the tool through the new growth from 3 o'clock towards 9 o'clock. Then, pull the tool down until it stops at the beginning of the lock at the new growth line of demarcation. The line of demarcation for locks is the point where the new growth meets the lock. This is the starting point of the rotation. As the tool exits the left side of the head, towards the left ear, thread the end of the lock through the tool:

- If the tool is a 2.5 inch hair pin push the end of the lock through the U-shaped tip.
- If the tool is a crochet needle, make sure the hook *and* the latch is all the way on the other side, the hair will be secured inside of the hook and the door of the latch pushed shut, then pull the end of the lock through.
- If the tool is a form of latch tool the shape of a threading needle, push the end of the lock through the hole.

Once the end of the lock is secured inside of the latch tool, pull the end of the hair back out towards the right ear. If the locks are long enough, (longer than four inches) continue the latching rotation, leaving the end of the lock threaded inside of the latch tool[60]. If the locks are short, take the end of the lock out of the latch tool and continue with the latching rotation, by rethreading each time.

4th Rotation (Fig 5.5)
Enter at 6 o'clock position/ exit and thread or loop the lock at 12 o'clock position/pull out at 6 o'clock position

Enter from the direction of the shoulder region, the 6 o'clock point along the head, the tip of the tool enters the loose new growth on the lower side of the head. The shoulders are the reference point. Push the tool through the new growth from 6 o'clock towards 12 o'clock at the top of the head. Then, pull the tool down until it stops at the beginning of the lock at the new growth line of demarcation. The line of demarcation for locks is the point where the new growth meets the lock. This is the starting point to begin the rotation. As the tool exits the top side of the head, thread the end of the lock through the tool:

- If the tool is a 2.5 inch hair pin push the end of the lock through the U-shaped tip.
- If the tool is a crochet needle, make sure the hook *and* the latch is all the way on the other side, the hair will be secured inside of the hook and the door of the latch pushed shut, then pull the end of the lock through.
- If the tool is a form of latch tool the shape of a threading needle, push the end of the lock through the hole.

Once the end of the lock is secured inside of the latch tool, pull the end of the hair back out towards 6 o'clock. If the locks are long enough, (longer than four inches) continue the latching rotation, leaving the end of the lock threaded inside of the latch tool[61]. If the locks are short, take the end of the lock out of the latch tool and continue with the latching rotation, by rethreading each time. If the last latch is within an eighth of an inch to the scalp, stop and move on to the next lock. Latching is a skill that can be learned and can be mastered. There are mistakes that may be made

---

[59]If the tool is a crochet needle, the end of the lock will need to be threaded at each loop point. If it's a tool with a hole, continue the threading rotation continuously.

[60]If the tool is a crochet needle, the end of the lock will need to be threaded at each loop point. If it's a tool with a hole, continue the threading rotation continuously.

[61]If the tool is a crochet needle, the end of the lock will need to be threaded at each loop point. If it's a tool with a hole, continue the threading rotation continuously.

along the way; however, can be corrected within reason. Please take note of the 'Do Not list' for latching with respective corrective measures.

Do Not!

1. Do Not! Latch too tightly at the base of the lock!

If a hard bump is felt on the scalp at the base of the lock with or without a white top, it is too tight! Just like braids that are too tight, the white tip and knot is the follicle and the follicle houses the living part of the hair strand, the papilla. If the papilla is damaged or removed, due to stress, it can result in traction alopecia, which occurs from tension due to hairstyles and chemical damage. Traction alopecia is reversible in some cases, in many, it is not. Traction alopecia can be avoided by leaving an eighth of an inch of loose hair at the base of the lock after tightening. This is why it is so important to have a full rotation of new growth before tightening the roots. Usually an eighth of an inch is easy to leave if there's enough new growth to create a four point rotation. If hair is latched too tightly, the hair can be loosened, by saturating with water. Place scalp under the force of water to loosen, massage fingers at the scalp under the force of the water. Ibuprofen will lessen the pain. Do not pull the lock tightly through the hole. Once the hair strand goes through the base of the lock, it is latched. The hair is forgiving; but, the root-bed is not! In some cases, the hair can become susceptible to breakage. It will depend on the health of the hair strand.

2. Do Not! Latch through the same hole more than once!

This may occur if the new growth has more than one rotation of tightening and because of a growth spurt during the normal four to six week period, or a lapse in the tightening schedule. When beginning the second round of rotations, enter to the right of the original point of entry. Imagine a clock. If the clock position was 12 o'clock on the 1st rotation, on the second rotation, enter at 1 o'clock. If the 2nd position on the first rotation was 3 o'clock, enter at 4

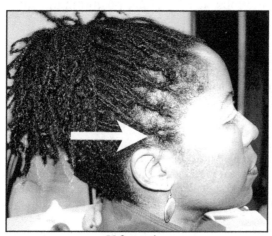

Y-formation

o'clock on the 2nd position of the second rotation and so on. Continue in this fashion until the hair is tightened within an eighth of an inch away from the scalp. Never latch through the same hole more than once. If the latch tool is entered in the same hole, the result can be a Y-formation or a hole in the locks. A Y-formation is when the hair distinctly separates into two separate parts, forming a Y along the scalp. A hole and a Y-formation are both resolved by repeating a latch to the right of the original point of insertion.

If holes remain along the lock shaft, sew the hole closed by using a thread that resembles the hair color and sew the hole shut until it's not seen. Tie a knot and clip the ends of the thread. This will erase the hole. If there's no more new growth to latch, remember to start the next retightening section to close the hole. For example, this picture shows a letter Y-formation as the first lock along the hairline above the left ear. Close the Y-formation by inserting the latch tool from north to south, across the top of the Y formation. The Y-formation will close. It's not okay to repetitively enter through the same hole. The locks would become weak and fragile from the holes.

3. Do Not! Pull loose hairs from other root-beds!

Sometimes locks will join together by accident. This happens frequently with the crochet hook, which has a tendency to snag adjacent hairs from other locks. If the root-beds from locks are inadvertently latched together, try to push the lock out through the same hole. Gently try to locate the hole and try to work the lock that doesn't belong out through the same hole, in the opposite direction it was pulled through. Prevent this from occurring by securing the neighboring locks out of the way with a duck-billed clipped.

4. Do Not! Latch dry hair!

Latching hair that is dry weakens the lock by compromising the root-bed. Always latch on damp hair. Keep hair damp by spritzing with the healthy hair growth spritz.

DO!

1. Do! Pull the lock all the way through the hole!

Once the length of the lock comes through the hole, continue until the hair is pulled through the hole all the way! Interlocking the hair is like threading a needle. Do not pull the hair so tightly that it breaks. Once the lock goes through the base of the lock, it is latched. Proper tension is critical, if the latch feels like a knot, loosen the latch by spritzing and pressing down on the knot, pinching the knot between the fingers, it will smooth out. The hair is forgiving. In some cases, the hair can become susceptible to breakage. It depends on the health of the hair strand.

2. Do! Pull loose and stray hairs into the lock. There are two key ways to do this:
  a. Finger Twirl
- With thumb and index finger, place a dime sized amount of pre-made healthy hair growth gel between the two fingers and massage down the length of the damp lock.
- Wrap dampened lock around the index finger and twirl the lock from the root-bed to the end of the lock.
- This method is helpful during the first year of locking as the lock develops. It's not noticeable until after six or more consecutive months of locking.

  b. Latch the loose hairs into the lock[62]
- Instead of threading the end of the lock into the latch tool, pull the loose hairs through the lock with latch hook. The latch hook tool is especially helpful, because it loops around the loose hair and pulls the loose hairs through the lock.
- Pull the loose, stray hair through the lock with the latch tool.
- This can be done during the tightening of the root-bed and down the length of the lock, as needed. The purpose is to secure those stray hairs.
- If locker prefers an extra neat look, follow with finger twirl, sealed with pre-made healthy hair growth gel.

3. Do! Roll only damp hair!

4. Do! Use a healthy nourishing gel!

5. Do! Roll every four to six weeks!

---

[62]If it's a crochet needle, the end of the lock will need to be threaded at each loop point. If it's a tool with a hole, continue the threading rotation continuously.

CREATING BEAUTIFUL LOCKS ON A DIME!

Let's Roll!
Tightening The Lock Foundation
by

Palm-Rolling($$)

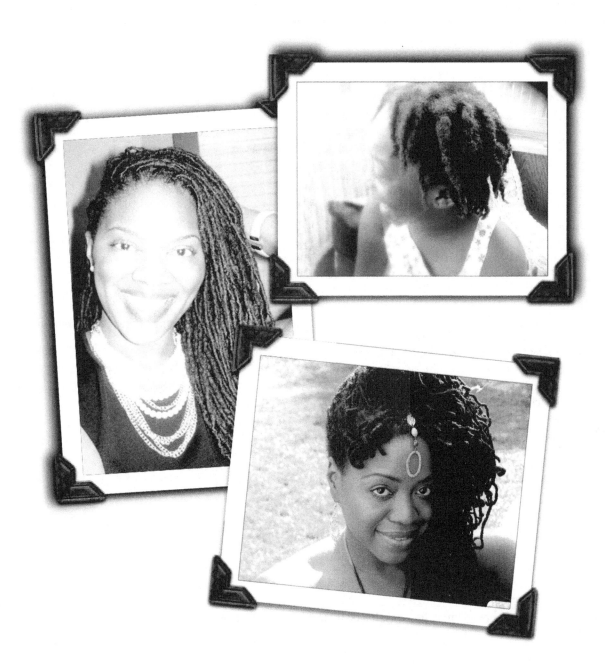

Palm-rolling to tighten locks is the traditional way to maintain locks, incorporating loose and stray hairs into the lock by twisting the roots, then smooth the length of the lock shaft to the end. It is a temporary way to tighten the new growth, attached to the lock. This method automatically gives a cylindrical shape to the lock. Palm-rolling directs the intertwined hairs that will become the lock, into a direction that encourages transformation, as the locking process matures. It's simple and easy to do. Unlike interlocking, which requires technical skills and does not automatically incorporate stray, loose hairs, palm-rolling is relatively simple. The hardest thing to remember is which direction to consistently tighten the lock. The locks can be palm-rolled or twisted clockwise or counterclockwise. Make a note of the direction in the lock chart and consistently tighten the lock in the direction of the installed foundation. This pattern of tightening will last up to two weeks if the hair is not disturbed. The disadvantage is keeping the hair in this pattern, because it unravels easily. The process of matting for the first time can take from three to six months, it may take longer for wavy, straight hair textures. Lockers that have busy lifestyles that involve frequent hair washing, exercise or a meticulous or self-conscious personality, may have challenges with this technique. This technique works best with Type 3, 4 hair textures. Type 1 and Type 2 lockers can palm-roll with gel[63] after the 2-step twist combination method, to further secure a cylindrical shape. Always palm-roll the roots, twisting can lead to uneven tension at the line of demarcation and breakage in the future.

Personality:

- Confident
- Patient, locks will unravel and expand

Who?

- Anyone with patience!
- Corporate employee
- Student with carefree personality
- Traditional locker
- Artistic personality

Texture:

- Tightly coiled hair texture
- All hair textures: Type 1, 2, 3, 4

Skill Set:

- Medium skill level required. No tool required, only hands
- Can be combined with latching for a distinct look desired at the hairline

Result:

- Neat look when first tightened. Hair expands and unravels from moisture. Can take months to lock, depending upon hair texture.
- Plump, full locks may appear cylindrical

Advantage:

- Defined look when first tightened
- Quick, 30 minutes to four hours on average, depends on lock size and partings
- Looks like locks quickly

Disadvantage:

- Locking agent
- Unravels easily
- Many experience build up, but not all

---

[63]Pomades can lead to build up in the locks. It's better to latch straighter hair textures, then palm-roll with the healthy hair growth gel (Type 1, 2, 3).

How to Palm-Roll

Let's Roll!

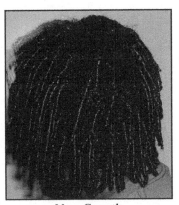

New Growth

1. Place a quarter size amount of pre-made Nourishing Conditioning and Holding Gel in the palm of the hand and spread gel inside of palms evenly.
2. Place the lock between the palms of the hand and roll the lock from the base to the end of the lock.
3. Roll the right hand down the left hand palm until the fingertips of the right hand come down to the base of the left palm.
4. Lay the lock down against the scalp. The lock can be secured with clips or twisted into a style to hold.
5. Air dry or dry under cool air to dry locks.
6. Massage a light oil onto locks once dry.

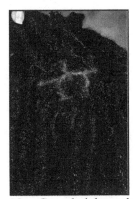

New Growth tightened by palm-rolling

Do!

1. <u>Do!</u> Roll only damp hair!

2. <u>Do!</u> Use a healthy nourishing gel!

3. <u>Do!</u> Roll every four to six weeks!

4. <u>Do!</u> Roll the hair the same direction every time!

Do Not!

1. <u>Do Not!</u> Palm-roll or twist on dry hair. Hair must always be damp from a fresh wash, preferably, or spritz with the healthy hair growth juice.

2. <u>Do Not!</u> Palm-roll or twist the roots more than once every four to six weeks no matter how puffy, or frizzy the roots get!

3. <u>Do Not!</u> Use hydrophobic hair products: waxes, pomades[64]!

4. <u>Do Not!</u> Color the locks without the care of a trained natural hair professional!

---

[64]Just Say No! Ingredients listed in The Holistic Hair Care Chapter.

CREATING BEAUTIFUL LOCKS ON A DIME!

Not-**Tightening The Lock Foundation**
by
Free-form/Semi-Free Form ($0.00)

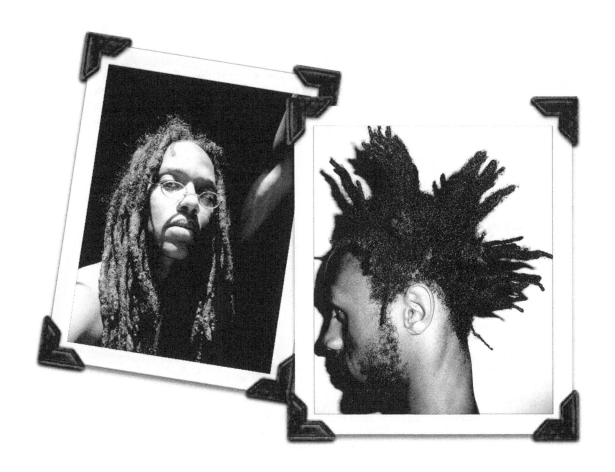

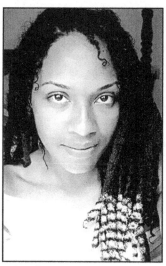

Semi-Organic Free-formed beauty

Free-forming

Free-forming is the simplest way to maintain locks. The only maintenance involved is washing the locks and keeping the scalp clean. Free-forming can be done straight from organic locks, which are simply locks that are formed by washing the hair and letting it uniquely clump, without intervention. Free-forming can also be performed on locks that have been previously maintained and tightened. When free-forming, there is no popping the root-bed. Locks are allowed to form at will.

Semi-free forming

Semi-free forming is another low maintenance tightening technique to maintain locks. Unlike free-forming, semi-free forming involves separation of the root-beds of adjacent locks by popping. Semi- free-forming can be done from locks that have been previously maintained and tightened, or from locks that have been organically created. Locks that are tightened only 1-3 times/ year are also considered semi-free formed locks. The only maintenance involved is washing the locks and keeping the scalp clean, and separating the roots by popping them.

Organic-Free Forming

To organically free-form, it's important to avoid product use and manipulation of the hair. The hair is allowed to form and grow without intervention. There are variations of organic free-formed locks. For example, some may free-form installed locks organically, after installation. Others may grow organic locks, then decide to tighten the roots by semi-free forming. Organic locks require the highest level of maturity and restraint, patience and the least amount of attention.

Personality:
- Tender-headed
- Confident
- Flexible, not controlling
- Prefers not to do his/her hair

Who?
- Musician/Artist
- Retired

Skill set:
- Lowest technique skill set required
- No maintenance/ low maintenance

Texture:
- Best for Type 3, 4
- All textures can freeform once locks have matted and locked
- Loose look, carefree look, may look unkempt to some
- All can freeform or semi-free form after hair is locked

Advantage:

- No maintenance or low maintenance!
- No time! Just go!
- Independent of Stylist!
- No product!
- No tools!
- 100% self-maintenance

Disadvantage:

- Hair freely grows and shapes on its own
- Unkempt appearance, offensive to some, beautiful to others

CREATING BEAUTIFUL LOCKS ON A DIME!

Tightening The Lock Foundation
for
Sisterlocks™/Brotherlocks™
($$$$$)

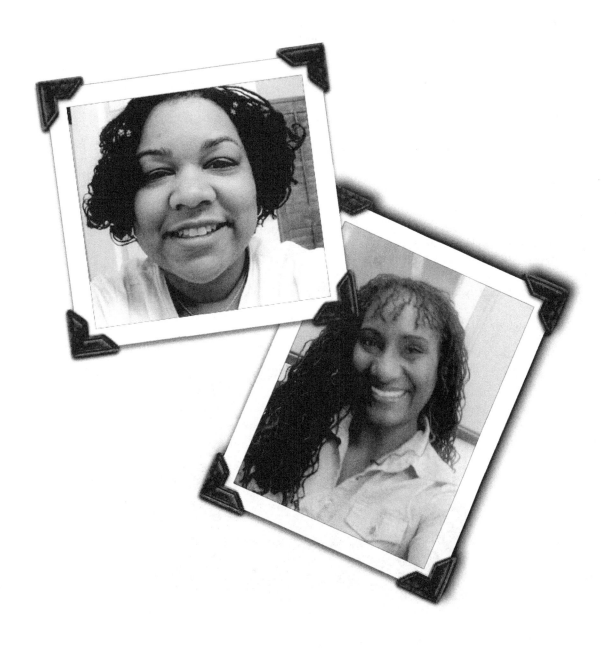

Sisterlocks™/Brotherlocks™

These microlocks are tightened with a special patented tool. Hair can be virgin, natural or chemically processed with two to four inches of new growth. Must be maintained by a certified Sisterlocks™ consultant. There is an option for client re-tightening certification. Please consult the Sisterlocks™ website at www.sisterlocks.com.

Personality:
- Those who have Sisterlocks™ and Brotherlocks™

Who?
- Those who have Sisterlocks™ and Brotherlocks™

Skill Set:
- Highly skilled, highly maintained with special products, tool and certified consultant
- Tightening class certification or done by Sisterlock™ consultant
- Go to www.sisterlocks.com for more information

Texture:
- See a certified Sisterlock™ consultant
- All, best with highly textured hair

Advantage:
- Aesthetic preference
- Successfully installed on chemically processed hair
- No product required
- Has been called microlocks
- Recognized program designed to produce entrepreneurs

Disadvantage:
- Time to retighten three to six hours, depends on size, partings, skill level of consultant
- Access to consultant may be limited
- Expense of learning self-maintenance

Result:
- Thin locks, tightly knit together with varying degrees of texture unique to each individual locker.

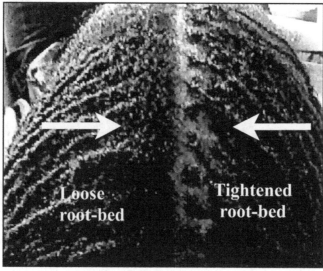

Untouched Sisterlock™ roots versus
tightened roots

Tightening The Lock Foundation
by
2-Step Twist Combination

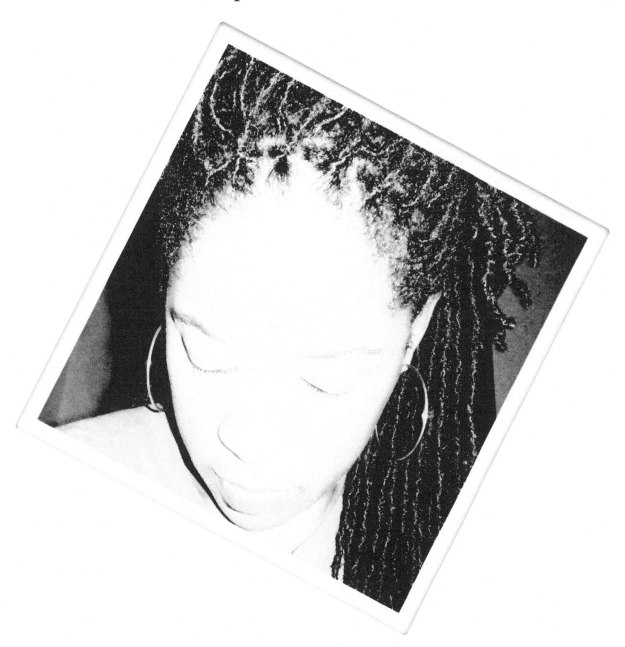

The 2-Step Twist Combination involves pinching the loose root-bed with the thumb and index finger, then turning the new growth in the direction of the lock formation with a preparation gel. As the root-bed is pinched, with each quarter turn, the new growth is latched. The advantage of this process is a neat, distinct root-bed with appearance of the palm-rolled locks that have been freshly rolled; yet, it is set in place by interlocking and will not unravel. When using this technique, each quarter twist is a new latch entry point. Be aware of the Y-formations[65], and insert into new entry points along the new growth to maintain strong locks.

Personality:
- Any

Who?
- Anyone interested in a distinct, secure root-bed
- Those particular about a freshly done appearance

Skill set:
- Skilled in combining and alternating between twisting and latching in a rotation

Texture:
- All

Result:
- A defined look that does not unravel

Advantage:
- Distinct, secure look

Disadvantage:
- High skill set high
- Product preferred

How to do the 2-Step Twist Combination:

1. Twist the hair by turning the wrist in the direction of the lock, either clockwise or counterclockwise.
2. After a quarter turn hold the twist with one hand, and latch to secure.
3. Continue with the quarter twist, hold, latch process until the root-bed is tightened within an eighth of an inch to the scalp.
4. Finger twirl or palm-roll down the length of the lock.
5. Place locks under a dryer set to cool or no heat.

---

[65]See The Root of The Matter

6

The Evolution of a Lock

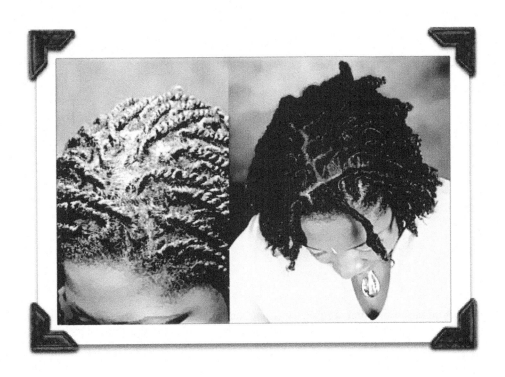

The purpose of the first year of locking is to lay a solid foundation for the maturing lock. Locking requires a series of changes, that seem long and tedious; however, in the grand scheme of this permanent process, the transformation time is quick and purposeful. The gestation period of a lock takes approximately twenty-four months[66]. For over 365 days, the hair will frizz, tangle, bud, knot, mat, shrink, expand, shed, condense, bunch, creep, unravel and crawl, until it reaches maturity to form locks. For many days, afterwards, the locks will continue to mature and shift from transforming to growing and tightening along the shaft of the lock. The process may not be the same for each locker; however, there are occurrences common to each phase of the transformation. Every lock will go through stages of infancy/pre-lock, teenage/budding, and maturity before becoming seasoned locks. Every hair strand will continue to cycle through the anagen, catagen, telogen phases, individually. On a microscopic level, each hair strand is made up of millions of DNA strands, carrying the same genetic instructions in tiny little cells that make up each hair fiber. Every phase and stage is interdependent upon the health of the individual, one another, outside influences and the DNA instructions. These traits are unique to each person, as the timing and longevity of these changes are guided under the direction of genetic design. The locking process requires commitment. Webster defines commitment as keeping a promise. Reliable. Dedicated. Unchanging. And this defines the mission that is required to grow a healthy head of locks. Assessing the journey in three developmental stages is key to transforming the mind, and accepting the locking process.

Developmental Lock Process

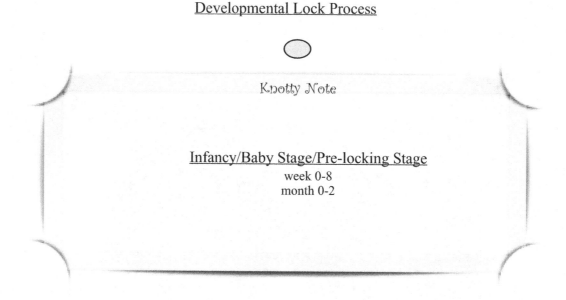

Knotty Note

Infancy/Baby Stage/Pre-locking Stage
week 0-8
month 0-2

Feelings:

Euphoria, excitement and determination are usually strong during this phase. There may be a sense of denial. The new locker may believe that his/her locks will uniquely continue to look neat and shiny. The hair style is temporary and by week three or four, it's important to seek encouraging pictures and support, because the hair will begin to frizz and look messy.

The infancy of the lock-evolution occurs during the first few weeks of the journey, lasting from month zero to two. The first half of the infancy stage (weeks zero through four) begins with a beautiful hair style also known as the

---

[66]See the chart at the end of this chapter on locking seasons.

installation foundation. It is difficult for many lockers to make it past the infancy stage, because they are dependent upon a neat presentation. By week four, the neat hair style is gone and the hair begins to clearly look disheveled as the process of frizz and shrinkage takes over. Because the cuticle of the highly textured hair comprises only 10-15% of the hair strand, 90% of it behaves like the cortex: soft, pliable, moldable, frizzing and shrinking because of the elastic behavior and porosity of the hair. Porosity is a measurement of the amount of moisture absorbed by the hair. About 35% of the hair's strength is due to millions of hydrogen bonds. Salt bonds comprise another 35% of the hair's composition. Salt bonds help to organize the protein chains. Salt and hydrogen bonds are weak bonds, broken easily by water. Consequently, if there is moisture in the air, or the hair gets wet, it will easily revert to its natural spiral formation, with potential energy conserved within the springs of the coil, causing the hair to expand and shrink and mat easily, forming knots and tangles, which is the evidence of this movement.

Straight, wavy hair textures must be forced to mat. By week four, straight, wavy hair textures may exhibit shrinkage, as the manual manipulation of backcombing helps to lift the cuticles and make the hair more porous. Remember, week four is the point where the hair style stays or the locking process begins, and marks the time to tighten the new growth at the root-bed as the shape of the future lock evolves, as the lock formation takes shape.

Because of the porosity of the hair, the hair will frizz. Frizz must be embraced, because it is an essential step along the locking process! It is the first telltale sign that the hair's matrix system is locking. For a highly textured locker, one of the hardest things to embrace is the frizz. The frizz arrives and may depart inconspicuously. Highly textured hair may form a halo of frizz around the locks for months, years. When the frizz comes and when the frizz goes depends on the texture of the hair. Many will see changes after the first year, as the frizz subsides for many lockers. There are hair styles and techniques that can be implemented to minimize the frizz; but, the frizz never truly goes away[67]. There is hope! Frizz can be reduced with hydration! Nourish the hair with hydration from the inside out! Drink more water, and feed the hair moisture rich ingredients, not products laden with petroleum and mineral oils. For optimal results, seal in that moisture with an emollient based product(also known as a heavy oil)[68].

After frizzing, comes shrinkage. Shrinkage occurs, because the hydrophilic bonds in the hair are highly cohesive and like to stick together. The elasticity of highly textured hair can range from 20-80%, depending upon hair texture. If pulled, healthy hair can expand up to 50% when wet and up to 20% ,when dry[69]. This occurs because the water composition in the hair is 90%! The more highly textured, the greater the elasticity, the greater the shrinkage. As discussed in The State of the Hair Chapter, elasticity creates movement along the lock. Elasticity is measured by tensile strength. Tensile strength measures the tension that can be applied before the hair breaks. The State of the Hair Chapter explores this trait with the tensile strength test to assess elasticity. Very poor tensile strength means hair is prone to damage and breakage.

---

[67]The Lock Challenge Chapter.

[68]The Holistic Hair Care Chapter.

[69]Salon Fundamentals: a Resource for Your Cosmetology Career. Evanston, IL: Pivot Point International, 2000. Print.

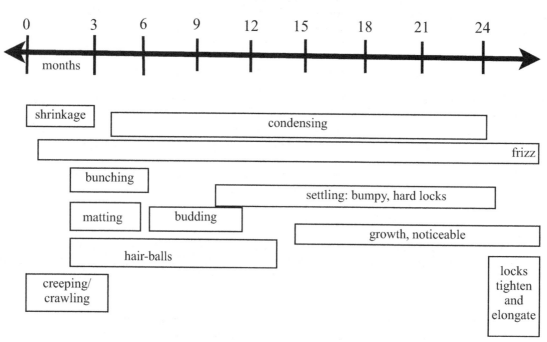

Fig. 6.1 Monthly timeline of the lock transformation process.

To restore the elasticity of dry hair, hydrate from the inside out. Daily intake of water should be equal half the body weight. A 100 lb person, should drink 50 oz in water. Feed the hair follicles moisture rich ingredients such as Organic Aloe Vera juice spritzes, seal with an emollient and cover the hair at night with a satin scarf. Highly textured hair begins to settle after month forty-eight, with frizzing and shrinkage occurring interchangeably leading to the condensing process. Straight hair, cuticle rich hair, only condenses because it is forced to mat from backcombing. Straight hair will settle instead of shrink. Settling is an important part of the infancy stage of straight hair, because settling is required for straight hair to begin to tangle, mesh, intertwine and knot up, forming the core of the future lock. When locks are 'settled', it simply means that they won't unravel on their own because the locking process has begun. As the hair frizzes and shrinks, hairs along the root-beds of adjacent locks begin to crawl and creep. Crawling/creeping/marrying is the process of other strands sticking to hair strands of another root-bed. This phenomena may be noticeable around week eight. Week eight marks the second tightening session and for the first time, the locks may need to be separated at the root-base. Some locks may unravel and hair that has not been properly cared for between washings, at the root-base, may be matted for the first time. Keep the scalp clean and separated for a successful journey from this point onward. Any or all of these activities may continue to occur throughout the locking process, from this point onward, as locks thicken, harden and condense.

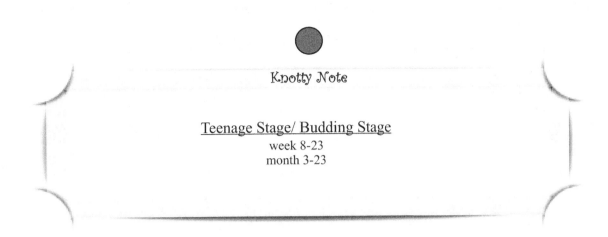

Knotty Note

Teenage Stage/ Budding Stage
week 8-23
month 3-23

Feelings:

Frustration sets in as the soft, pliable locks begin to harden. The frizz may become a major concern. The condensing process begins with unsightly buds. There's a new adjustment to deal with as the locking process envelopes the installation hairdo. Anxiety may set in as the locker realizes that the hair is locking. Concern and nervous anxiety captures the mood of this stage as the excitement of the locking process commences. Awkward teenage insecurities may arise, and the locker may feel shy and hesitant about going out in public. It's important not to control the hair with accessories and gels. The babies are growing up, and developing a mind of their own. Let them grow freely. Frustration mounts as they are less controllable. Psychologically, this stage can be difficult. This stage can test the most patient of souls and cause a type A personality to run for the chemical relaxer. Seek support and encouragement! This is just a phase; and, this too shall pass!

Physical:

The physical line between the teenage stage and the adult stage gets blurry and the methodologies out there vary. The second half of the teenage stage is very different from the infancy stage, and very different from the adult stage, just like middle school children are neither teens nor adults, but caught in an awkward in between stage. During the second half of the teenage stage, roughly months thirteen to twenty-three, the locks will begin to show growth while they continue to condense. During the teenage stage, the locks may appear unattractive to the locker. The hair continues to defiantly do what it wants to, including going off in different directions than originally positioned. Wearing hair styles that emphasize curl textures such as braid-outs and curls, while setting with organic Aloe Vera gel can give the hair a presentable appearance, while transitioning through the difficult teenage months, minimizing the differences. Also encourage the locker to focus on beautiful lock pictures, to get through this bumpy stage. Until the magic lock moment occurs, encourage the locker to blog about the journey, take pictures and copious notes to document the update. The babies will grow to become teenagers that become adults. Having the pictures to reflect upon will be a wonderful reminder of how far the locks have come, as time moves along.

As the hair style continues to disappear, the teenage stage will continue anywhere from week eight to month twenty-three. The new growth at the root-bed and loose hairs along the lock continue to cross over into different sections, creeping and meshing among adjacent locks as the manicured parts continue to fill in with new growth and loosened hair. The inner matrix begins to form as loose hair begins to align along the shaft of the lock, often in the middle, forming a structure that will be called a bud. The inner matrix is the foundation of each lock. It starts with a bud, of shed hair, the hair gathers, forming the nucleus of the bud, transforming into the nucleus of the lock. From this point, the bud reaches in both directions, directing the foundation to transform into a network of matted hair. The frizzing process and the shrinkage process progress. Bunching may be the precursor to the pea sized knot or bubble along the lock shaft that will become known as a bud for many months. Bunching can occur from:

- A straight texture (can cause hair to unravel and tangle unevenly)
- Overuse of conditioning products during the early stages of locking
- Washing hair without banding
- Coloring the hair after locking

In some cases, bunching can be a natural step before the pea sized bud forms, or it can occur in addition to budding and can be reversed[70]. Mature bunching can add character to a lock. It is a matter of preference whether to 'fix' a bunched lock. Budding and bunching are different. Budding is more of a defined circular mass that hardens, bunching is an undefined 'bunch' of hair that meshes together with no clear nucleus. It may not get hard and there may be holes inside the bunched lock, as opposed to buds. Buds are usually hard masses of hair centralized along the lock.

The frizz, shrinkage, movement, bunching, budding and shedding give way to condensing. The difference between shrinkage and condensing is the texture of the lock. Condense means to make more dense or compact; reduce the volume or extent, concentrate. The concentration of something is the thickness, the density. A condensed lock is stiff and compact. When locks are in the process of shrinking, they are soft and simply reduce to over half of their size. Shrinkage, growth cycle, washings, tightenings and time give way to shedding. Shed hairs release from the follicle and fill up the inner matrix expanding in volume, forming a soft net. The inner matrix in the lock core captures the dead hair that disperses from the scalp. Some of the hair released will be hair with the bulb attached. This is the papilla released from the follicle, which provides the source of nutrients for the growing hair strand. The net will condense into a hard mass, known as the bud. The bud will become the nucleus of the lock. From this matrix, the hair will begin to intertwine, mesh and reach up and down solidifying the core of the lock foundation, transforming the original matrix with what will become known as locks, giving the instructions to all new growth to join in the locking process. The bud forms at the older section of the lock. The older part of the lock will continue to condense tightly and mature. To discern between bunching and budding, the rule of thumb is to always wait for the bud to form along the lock shaft, that way a budding bud will never be disturbed inadvertently.

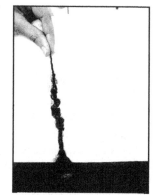

A lock in the process of condensing.

As the installed foundation condenses, the length of the locks become noticeably shorter. The locks will shorten by condensing as they spin and intertwine into cylindrical units along the lock, prompted by the coiled formations. They expand, hardening outward from the core as the lock swells from the shed hair that has increased in volume, compacted and condensed into a larger lock. They become hard as the texture changes becoming less consistent along the lock. The locks take on a fuzzy halo and may have a grey appearance, especially in photographs, as the sheen disappears from the hair style. This is normal. The locks are very bumpy, uneven and may be unappealing to the locker.

Shed hair continues to work its way down the length of the lock. The shed hair that is not caught in the inner matrix, extends down the length of the lock to become the sealed tip of the lock. Once sealed, the matrix is locked in and the lock continues to evolve. Some shed hair may fall off from the tip of the lock. They look like tiny balls of hair dangling off the end of the lock, and are known as hair-balls. They are most noticeable after washing the hair. If a loose, curly look is desired, at the end of the lock, pull the hair ball. If not, it's best to not disturb the locking process with pulling, no matter how much they dangle off the lock. Some locks will never seal. Sealed locks have rounded tips that are compact and tightly knitted into a closed tip[71]. Other locks have loose curl spirals that resist sealing and locking. Once the shaft of the lock is locked, the loose curl spiral can be left or snipped off. However, based upon the hair texture, some locks will always unravel at the end, forming loose curl spirals. How the hair-balls form is dependent upon the hair texture, which is dictated by the DNA.

---

[70]Go to The Lock Challenge Chapter to see a visual of bunching and budding.

[71]The Lock Challenge Chapter

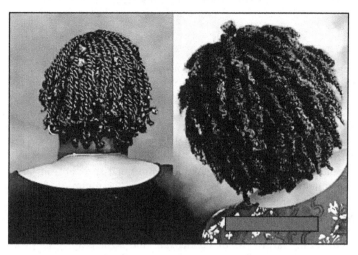

The transformation process is amazing!

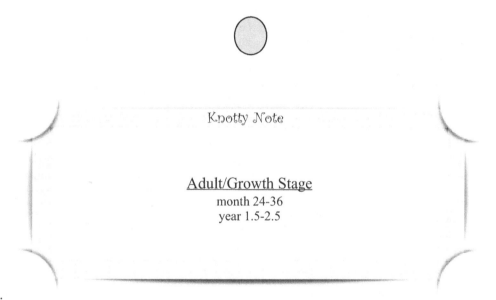

Knotty Note

Adult/Growth Stage
month 24-36
year 1.5-2.5

Feelings:

The difficult part of the journey is almost over. Now, the journey is referred to in the terms of months, instead of weeks. Relief and let down might take over. Many don't realize the amount of energy expended during the first twenty-three months. Because hair growth is not noticeable, a locker may feel frustrated and sad. Growth will come during the second half of the teenage stage around month thirteen. If the hair was locked with greater than four inches of length, the locker experiences an enormous setback with shrinkage first, then condensing, creating thicker locks with significantly less length. The locker with short hair, shorter than two inches, now has locks the length of the longer-haired locker. There is virtually no difference[72]. The locks might be thinner, as well. This can lead to enormous frustration. For the long-haired locker, anticipate this variance and embrace the process. It takes much more energy for long hair to transform than short hair to grow into locks and the price to pay is length, for the first thirteen months. The hard part is over! Now, it's time to wait and grow!

---

[72]The Lock Challenge Chapter

locks and the price to pay is length, for the first thirteen months. The hard part is over! Now, it's time to wait and grow!

Physical:

During months zero through thirteen, the growth may not be visible because the hair is busy cycling through the process of, frizzing, shrinkage, condensing, shedding, bunching, budding, and expansion. Finally, the activity of lock transformation is slowing down and the locks tighten. Tightening of the lock is the latter stage of condensing, the precursor is shrinkage. As locks mature, first they shrink, then condense, then expand outwardly. Upon maturity, they tighten and become tighter and uniform. The hair is always in a cycle of growth, rest and shedding. In fact, besides frizz, the shedding of hair is another signal which alerts the locker that the process is indeed progressing through the necessary cycles. When hair bulbs are visualized along the shaft of the lock, the brief telogen phase has kicked out another hair strand, making room for a new hair strand that sprouts from the root. The anagen phase, is predetermined by genetic precursors and lasts from two years, to a maximum of six years. When the adult stage is reached, the length will slowly become visible as the older part of the lock continues to condense, become shorter and the new growth becomes the length of the lock. As the cellular division/mitosis process occurs inside the follicles, dead hair is pushed up and out through the scalp contributing to the new growth. Now, even though the lock is an adult, it must go through a process of condensing and tightening. This process normally ends around month twenty-three. The care of the new growth will determine the look of the mature lock as the older shaft, merges and the newer shaft continues to tighten and condense.

After the lock has hardened, it is solid, firm, and the ends are mostly sealed. If they have not sealed by this point, they usually won't. That's fine. As long as the shaft of the lock is firm, the lock has locked. Lock maturity is all about growth, and tightening; whereas, lock infancy is all about shrinking, condensing and budding. The wide, condensed lock that dominated the latter part of the teenage journey will now merge into a unique, more uniform lock that is tighter, more compact. There may still be a halo of frizz; but, it's usually less dominant now, than during the early months of locking. As lock maturity progresses, frizz usually disappears, or the locker becomes more accepting of it. Which one it is, is hard to tell. Some locks never loose their characteristic frizz; however, all locks can be groomed to minimize the frizz[73]. The annual celebration of the lock birthday, is usually met with hair-ball shedding for each lock-anniversary, henceforth.

The adult stage appears to be locked in the anagen stage because the hair will remain in a steady pattern of growth. However, any phase of the growth cycle can be occurring at any given time. Frizzing, condensing, tightening will continue along the older portion of the lock shaft. Subsequently, the new growth will continue to cycle through its own locking process while integrating with the older portion. Any locks that are combined will also continue to cycle through all stages and phases of the locking process. The process is continual and dynamic, never static.

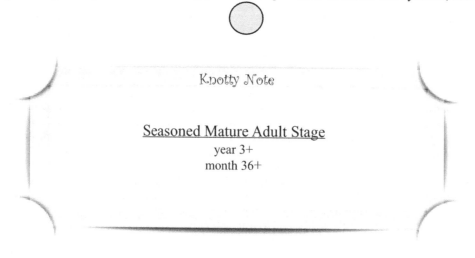

Knotty Note

Seasoned Mature Adult Stage
year 3+
month 36+

---

[73]The Lock Challenge Chapter

The second stage of the mature adult stage is the seasoned adult stage. This stage is characterized by new growth, tightening of the locks, annual shedding of the hair-balls at the end of the lock. The original lock has condensed until it is a 1-2 inch nub of hair that forms the tip of the lock, if latched for maintenance. If locks have been palm-rolled for maintenance, the tips may become thin and require trimming. The locks are uniform and may begin to shed, break at the ends, where the hair is the oldest. If the locks were installed from braids, the pattern may be visible. This is the area that was the original foundation, now a sealed or opened end. Locks are beyond mid-back. Locks will continue to contract into a tight matrix of cylindrical coils intermeshed inside of a networked matrix, thinning and elongating.

LOCK SEASONS		
WEEK	MONTH	LOCK STAGE
4	1	baby
8	2	baby
12	3	teen
16	4	teen
20	5	teen
24	6	teen
28	7	teen
32	8	teen
36	9	teen
40	10	teen
52	13	mature teen
92	23	mature teen
96	24	adult
144	36	seasoned adult

Lock Seasons

In summary, commitment is the ability to be true to a purpose, cause, self or others. Growing locks is about being true to self, in spite of the challenges that arise through the process. The process is not the end result, locks are the purpose. Staying focused on the product, locks, is the key to a successful locking journey. There really are locks on the other side of the buds, frizz and mess and they are beautiful. Acceptance and leaving the hair alone is the most challenging part of the journey. As a result, the process of locking is 90% mental and 10% physical.

Washing Dreaded
Locks of Hair

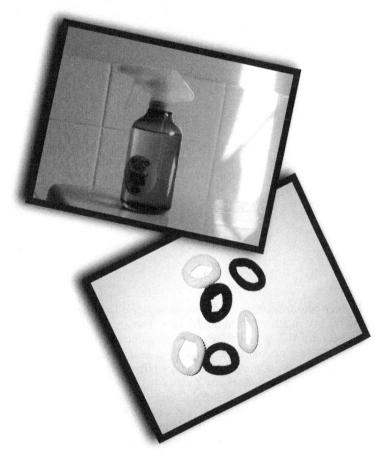

A common misconception is that locks cannot be washed clean and clear of dirt and debris. Or, that new locks should not be washed. How untrue! In fact, one of the best ways to wash highly textured loose and locked hair is in bundles of fortified strands that are secured to prevent tangling and matting during the washing process. The focus is on washing the scalp free of dirt and debris, while squeezing the soap through the hair. In addition, locks can be washed from day one! If locks are installed correctly, washing will not disrupt the locking process. If locks are washed incorrectly, they will still be clean and the hair will still develop into locks, with great character (non-uniform)! Locking is a process that thrives in perfect imperfections, making it hard to mess up. Remember that water is a lock's best friend, enhancing the locking process. Absolutely keep the scalp free of dirt, harmful bacteria and build up for good hygiene, health standards and thriving locks. For other reasons, licensed professionals may give other instructions. If the instructions differ, it's best to follow the stylist's instructions, because they are caring for the locks and usually have set bench marks and expectations that fall in line with given instructions. However, when a dirty scalp can not be tolerated, know that this chapter will serve as a point of reference of lock cleansing for all interested in clean hair.

Supplies for washing locks

1. Coated terry-bands
2. Hair net
3. Spray bottle or natural bar soap
4. Cotton, lent-free absorbent towels
5. Smooth and trim nails
6. Spray bottle
7. Micro-fiber towels/old T-shirt
8. Drain catcher
9. Natural bar soap/liquid shampoo
10. ACV rinse prepared in advance
11. Herbal Tea Conditioning rinse prepared in advance
12. Nourishing Conditioning gel prepared in advance

Directions

1. Prepare the Hair

It's important to prepare the hair before washing. Unlike loose natural hair, no laborious detangling sessions are required! However, preparing the hair in advance can troubleshoot bothersome issues that can arise later during lock development. Spray the scalp with the ACV pre-wash which helps to loosen dirt and sebum build-up. When washing immature coils, it's best to use a hair net or coated hair bands. For immature coils (baby locks), a stocking cap may be used. The hair net will confine the hair, limiting movement, while the hair is agitated in the washing process by water and soap, because baby coils are not yet solid and can easily unravel. For immature installation locks or any other type of installation that is maintained by palm-rolling, one of the main complaints is how quickly the hair unravels if the hair becomes wet, for any reason. A clever way to keep the twisted pattern at the roots in place is to secure the lock into banded sections with coated pony tail holders. This allows the pattern to remain and the locker to maintain a clean appearance in between the four to six week tightening. The bands and net do not need to be used on mature locks that have condensed and hardened. At this point, the mature locks have locked and the manipulation cannot disturb the installed lock; however, banding can become a viable alternative. If locking from braids, strand twists, Sisterlocks™/Brotherlocks™, locks can be braided into one big braid per section and secured with coated pony tail holders down the length of the lock-braid[74], this process is called banding. Make sure the ends are secured as well. This extra step will:

---

[74]See picture of banded braids prepped for washing.

1. Prevent bunching, slippage and unraveling
2. Focus on a clean scalp
3. Isolate the locks, by reducing manipulation
4. Efficiently cleanse locks and scalp

Some stylists may suggest cleansing the scalp with a cotton swab dabbed in astringent. That is a temporary solution until the hair can be thoroughly cleansed.

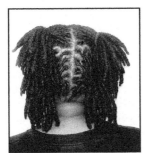

Locks gathered into sections
in preparation for washing.
A crucial step to reduce
developmental problems for
new locks that are palm-
rolled for maintenance.

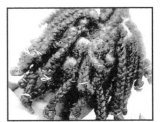

Locks gathered into their
braid sections and banded
in preparation for washing.

2. Prepare the Solutions

While oil and dirt is breaking down, prepare the hair solutions for washing. As discussed in the Holistic Hair Care Chapter, prepare the apple cider vinegar rinse, herbal tea conditioning rinse and nourishing spritz in advance. Natural bar soaps are excellent cleansers and moisturizers for all skin and hair purposes. Natural soaps such as true African Black Soap can be found in solid form or liquid. If African Black Soap or any other shampoo is used in liquid form, dilute it by adding a capful of soap to 8 oz of water in the spray bottle, Aloe Vera juice is a good option as well. Be sure to clean and trim the most important tools ahead of time, the hands. Smooth out nails, clipping and trimming away any jagged edges. Any snags on the nails will rip and tear the fragile hair. It's important to use a shampoo or a natural soap bar, not a conditioner, to wash locks[75].

---

[75]Holistic Hair Care Chapter

3. Spray and Wash

Now, that the hair is prepared and the preparations and supplies are gathered, begin spraying one section of the hair at a time. Whether the hair is in coils or mature, meticulously scrub the scalp with the pad of fingers, not nails. If the soap bar is used, lather the soap in hand and massage the soap into the scalp and scrub the scalp with ends of fingers as normal. Pump and squeeze the soap gently through locks until the warm water runs clear. Repeat for each section until the head is clean. Squeeze and pump the soap out of the hair with warm water.

4. Clarifying Post Rinse

Clarify the hair with the ACV mixture, an extra precaution, to ensure that soap and residue are completely out of the locks, proactively preventing build up. How often? As often as the locker desires to have soft, shiny locks free of soap residue. In fact, this step can also precede cleansing if hair is extremely dirty, to loosen up dirt and debris. Once again, spray each section, letting the ACV mixture penetrate the locks for three to five minutes. Then, rinse clear with warm water until the smell and the bubbles are gone. The final rinse should be with cold water. By then most of the ACV smell will be gone and the cold water will close the cuticles, leaving the hair shiny. Squeeze the water out of the hair and dry by squeezing the hair with the absorbent towel.

5. Conditioning Leave In

The leave in nourishing herbal tea conditioning rinse feeds the hair[76]. Leave it on the locks and don't rinse out! It will nourish the hair strand and the follicles, locking in moisture. Release locks and massage the mixture into the roots. If an alternative conditioner is substituted, make sure it is not of a cloudy consistency and low in oils and conditioners, unless locks are mature. If conditioning baby coils, leave the net on the hair, massaging the conditioner into the roots of the hair.

6. Drying the Hair

There are ways to dry locks without using damaging heat. Protecting highly textured hair from heat is crucial to protect the fragile bonds from breaking, leading to damaged hair[77]. To get extreme wetness out of the hair, drying with a micro-fiber towels or a cotton t-shirt is the first line of defense. Absorbent towels can be purchased from a local bed and beauty store, drug stores or health food stores. Place the towel around the head and squeeze the moisture out of the hair. An old cotton t-shirt is perfectly fine as well, and very budget friendly! The key is to use a towel or shirt that is free of lint! When the towel is completely saturated, repeat with a clean, dry towel.

When the weather is cold and time is pressing, hair can be dried with a blow dryer that has a setting for *no heat*. This setting uses room temperature air to blow at the hair. However, if time is available, air drying, naturally, is the best option for delicate locks. If styling, locks can always be wet set into a style, then allowed to air dry. When drying the hair, while it is still damp, it is important to pop the roots by separating any meshed root-beds that may have grown together during the growth or washing process. Some have successfully slept on wet locks by wearing a satin scarf covered with an absorbent towel. Others swear off sleeping on wet locks due to an increased chance of mildew build-up. Proactively rinsing the hair with ACV mixture is the first line of mildew prevention[78]. Once hair is dry, mature locks can be sealed with the nourishing hair oil for moisture and shine. If hair is still in the infancy stage, massaging a light oil such as jojoba oil is acceptable for the scalp. Do Not Rub the hair when drying, only gently squeeze with the towel.

---

[76]See The Holistic Hair Care Chapter.

[77]George, M. Michele. *The knotty truth: Managing Tightly Coiled Hair at Home*. 2nd ed. Columbus, Ohio: Manifest Publishing Enterprises, LLC 2007. Print.

[78]See The Lock Challenge Chapter.

Please, remember that good hygiene always comes first. Throw out those antiquated theories that locks should not be washed. Locks are hair and when hair is dirty, it needs to be washed, period!

Summary

1. Secure locks at the base with coated pony tail holders.
    • If locks are palm-rolled, make sure to secure the locks in the direction of the twist at the base of the lock[79].
    • Band groups of locks all the way to the ends if hair is long enough and not settled.
    • If locks are mature/settled, banding is not necessary.
    • Use a net for extremely immature locks.

2. Spray the scalp in one section with a dilution of shampoo and water.

3. Cleanse the scalp by scrubbing the scalp *only* with finger pads.

4. Pump and squeeze the soap carefully through the hair.

5. Rinse thoroughly with water.

6. Spray the Apple Cider Vinegar solution throughout the hair and let it sit for 1-2 minutes[80].

7. Rinse hair thoroughly with cool water.

8. With the absorbent towel, dry the hair by simply putting the towel on the head and squeezing out the water, DO NOT RUB THE HAIR!

9. Spray or massage in the Nourishing Conditioning rinse or gel into the hair and style or dry with a clean, dry towel.

10. Air dry is the healthiest way to dry the hair.

---

[79]See picture for demonstration on palm-roll sections for washing. For more instructions, see QoChemsit at http://www.youtube.com/watch?v=YkhlyLI8o7g.

[80]See The Holistic Hair Care Chapter.

CREATING BEAUTIFUL LOCKS ON A DIME!

8

Lock Challenges:
What to do
When, Why, How?

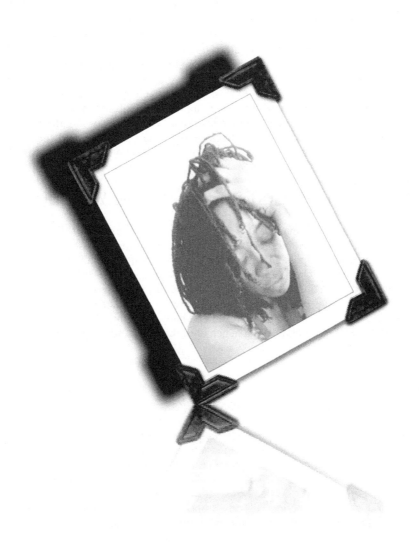

Help! My locks are thick and fat at the end and I can't get them through my tool to complete my rotation!

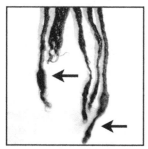

Common appearance of the original 12 inch latched-braid after 48 months.

This is a common problem for braidlocks, strand twists and some latched locks. The former installed foundation will shorten and condense to the end of the lock as a stub of its former glory. The hair that grows from the scalp is busy integrating and forming into a lock, while the installation foundation is busy, transforming. Remember, it takes longer for long hair to lock because of the laborious, time consuming and intricate process of integrating the new growth into the foundation 'lock', while the foundation lock attempts to mat and transform as well. The lock condenses lengthwise and compacts into a nub before tightening into a thinner lock. The latched root will become a long cord that is uniform in design, contrasting with the ends of the hair, noticeable around month twenty-four, extremely noticeable by year three and a half. The solution is to cut off the

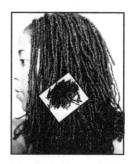

Month 49 the ends are cut away, leaving a smooth lock shaft. Never be afraid to cut in the name of healthy hair. It grows!

former braid or accept it. Many accept the size; however, cutting the former installed lock does take stress off of the roots. When the roots are stressed with the extra 'anchor' at the end of the lock, the root-base will constantly need to be combined to compensate for the weight. Palm-rolling may prevent the locks from forming bulky ends. It's very important to wait until months twenty-four to thirty-six before cutting away the former foundation at the end. At months twenty-four to thirty-six, the process of condensing is usually complete and the thick ends may not be noticeable until the elongation and the tightening processes is complete around month thirty-six. When this occurs, the end of the lock is noticeably thicker than the lock shaft.

Help! I cannot tell the difference between bunching and budding. What should I do about it?

The first thing to realize is that a bunch may become a bud. The second thing to realize is that any combining or unraveling of a lock will result in the locking process beginning anew, repeating itself. The third thing to recognize is that the final size of the portion manipulated will not be determined until months twenty-four through thirty-six. That means if locks are combined, picked apart, redone, the lock must cycle through the locking process from ground zero. With that in mind, sometimes it's difficult to distinguish budding from bunching. Lock bunching can occur at any point during the locking process. Bunching is often a precursor to budding, just not a prerequisite. Because budding blossoms during the teenage stage, it can end between months sixteen through twenty-four, it's not easy for an untrained eye to distinguish a bud from a bunch until then. Proactively prevent bunching by:

•Avoid oily products
•Band while washing the hair
•Avoid coloring until maturity
•Install an installation method that secures the hair texture

The cleansing process can contribute to bunching or budding as well, prevent this by banding locks in sections. Pay careful attention to massage the scalp. Squeeze the soap in a pumping motion through the locks. If the hair is palm-rolled or in coils, help stabilize the hair during shampoo time with a hair net to allow for manipulation with minimal lock movement.

Budding will naturally 'disappear' into the lock usually around month twenty-four. Bunching can add texture and uniqueness to a lock or it can be corrected. The following is a modified latching technique to close a bunched area along the lock:

1. Saturate the lock with a conditioning agent, press down and smooth out the area.
2. Begin latching from the bottom of the lock, towards the scalp with the crochet hook. Increase the number of latch rotations to secure the area tighter or braid tightly if the bunched area is at the end of the lock. If locks are palm-rolled, palm-roll the length of the lock.
3. Continue latching until the hole is sealed.

There's no right or wrong way to do this method, the goal is to tighten up the bunched area, minimizing expansion, reducing the bulk. As a result, the simple answer is to watch it. The solutions provided are only suggestions for those that are doing all the right things, but aren't ready to watch and wait.

Knotty Note

A trained eye can tell early on in the process and correct bunching. Bunching can occur from a loose texture, banding, slippage from excessive oily product use during the early months, or coloring locks after the lock installation.

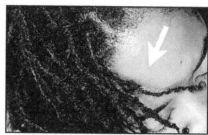

Budding or bunching? Only a trained eye can tell with touch and examination and careful observation.

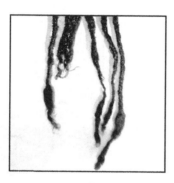
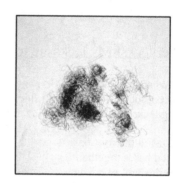

1st bunched ends taken apart at month 48 resulting in a normal amount of shed hair from the released bunch. Bunching can occur anywhere along the lock, but common for locks that are latched for maintenance.

Help! I have holes in my locks! What should I do?

Holes in locks are a result of improper latching and unique to tool locks. Simply 'sew' up the hole by inserting the tool through the hole by beginning the *next* latch insertion point to the side of the hole, closing it up. It is important to address this error because it can lead to lock breakage, if left unresolved.

Help! My locks are huge and I want smaller locks.

The first question to address is how old are the locks. At three years, or thirty-six months, locks just begin to mature. They thin out, become more uniform and truly hit a growth spurt. Latched locks will usually reduce in thickness by a half of their twenty-four month size. For example, stranded twists installed the size of a thick magic marker, latched for maintenance, may reduce down to a pencil sized lock by month thirty-six if interlocked. Palm-rolled locks reduce to a lesser extent. Biological traits such as density, porosity, texture, all play a roll in the final size of the lock. After month thirty-six (third lock anniversary), locks can be split to reduce their thickness. If locks are split before month thirty-six, the locks may be considerably smaller than the desired size, due to lock immaturity.

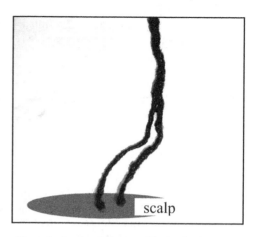

To make locks thinner, split the loose roots along the scalp. Make two separate branches. Latch the branches separately.

Splitting is the process of taking half of an inch to an inch of loose new growth and securing the sections separately, into two individual sections. This process can only be done on latched locks. Once separated, release one of the sections and begin latching from the lock portion down to the root. As the new growth continues to grow, continue latching separately[81]. As a Y-formation forms, growing longer, carefully cut the two arms apart at the intersection for a reduction in lock size.

Help! I want thicker locks! My locks are too thin!

Whether latched or twisted at the roots for maintenance, join the root-base of two adjacent locks to make them thicker. This is called combining. Combining locks can be performed many different ways:

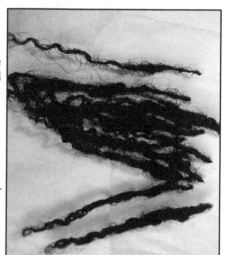

•Twist two locks together at the root-base.
•Latch adjacent root-bed bases together.
•Place rubber bands at the base of adjacent root-beds.
•Twist all the way to the end of the lock and palm-roll the locks together.
•Twist locks together and sew with a needle and thread to the end of the locks.
•Twist, latch, sew locks at the roots only.
•Latch at the roots and cut one of the branches.

Save the cut away pieces!

Cutting is best done under the watchful eye of a professional. The interwoven matrix is sometimes dependent upon the cut-away portion. Always save any part of the lock that is cut off for future emergencies! The thicker root base will create a larger lock. However, if both parts of the lock remain intact, after combining, an even larger lock is created, so choose the method carefully!

---

[81]See The Root of the Matter Chapter.

Help! Help me save my locks! The roots are thinning!

Thin roots are usually a result of tension placed on the root-base from the weight of the lock. The lock is heavy and pulls on the fragile follicles. When locks begin to bunch, bud and swell, root thinning will become evident. Combining the root-base of two adjacent locks, will strengthen the locks and the roots. Minimize the use of tension hairstyles and heavy accessories. Spray the roots daily with the nourishing spritz. Semi-free forming and free-forming are also excellent ways to strengthen the root-bed, giving it rest and a chance to recover. It's critical that the hair is only tightened every four to six weeks. Never twist or latch the hair more than every four to six weeks. This is mentioned many times throughout this book, because it is important. Excessive tightening of the new growth stresses the roots, weakening the whole area of the lock being tightened. Encourage the new growth to flourish with healthy massages. Massage a nourishing oil treatment into the roots and tie it down with a satin scarf at night.

In rare cases, thinning locks are from nervous hair tugging and pulling or medical conditions. Seek the help of a medical professional and look for lock caps that are sold to augment hair loss by adding lost locks to a weave cap, sewing them on, allowing the locker to wear their locks like a wig without detection.

Help! My hair is matting at the roots and sticking together!

It is important to pop the roots by spritzing and separating, gently. Popping can be done anytime, as long as the hair is slightly damp, after shampooing. Integrate popping into the post wash regimen to prevent matting. If extending tightening beyond four to six weeks, hair will easily mat. Find a maintenance routine that keeps up with maintenance sessions to prevent matting. Massage a nourishing oil treatment into the roots.

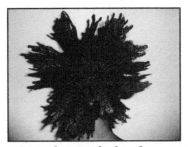

Matted roots of a free-former

Help! My hair is a frizzy mess, make it stop!

Frizz is one of the top complaints during the locking process. Unfortunately, frizz is necessary. If the hair is not frizzing, it is not locking. The first step is to embrace the frizz then put these good tips into practice. Find styles to reduce the frizz like braid-outs and twist-outs. Massage the nourishing gel into the locks and the roots, secure with a satin scarf to minimize frizz, leave on for at least ten minutes. Massage the nourishing gel and plait the locks to help minimize frizz. Smooth the nourishing gel with the index and middle fingers to the fragile temple hair to help tame frizzy edges and seal with castor oil, secure with a satin scarf for at least 15 minutes.

Grooming can also minimize frizz. Grooming is the process of trimming frizz off of the lock. This technique is best performed by a trained professional, if at all. Just like bunching, it's difficult to successfully tell what is frizz and what is hair that is needed in the locking process. Grooming is common for Sisterlocks/Brotherlocks™. For many, frizz will disappear with lock maturity. For many, frizz will never truly disappear, acceptance is truly peace of mind for a locker. Hydrating from the inside out and wearing braid-outs can reduce the 'appearance' of frizz.

Help! My hair smells like mildew!

Mildew can grow in locks from product build up and sleeping on moist locks. The ACV rinse helps to clarify the locks[82]. Be proactive! Some of the signs that locks may be breeding grounds for mildew:

•Locks look dry or dusty, even after washing many times
•Scalp is constantly itchy
•Un-normal hardening and stiffness of locks
•A damp smell
•Going to bed on damp locks

To prevent mildew, use clear conditioning products and minimize product build up by washing hair frequently. Cloudy conditioning products attract moisture but also can leave behind residue. When cleaning locks of mildew, it is important to clarify many times with the ACV rinse, as many times as it takes, until the smell is gone. If the ACV rinses do not work, escalate the process by soaking the locks in a bucket of soapy water for at least five minutes with a mixture of one part dish detergent to nine parts water. Squeeze out excess water and put on a shower cap for thirty minutes. Rinse. Repeat. Another solution is to spritz an astringent or witch hazel mixed with a couple of drops of tea tree oil, mixed 1:9, as well. Spray into hair, cover with a shower cap. Rinse out[83]. Follow up with a good moisturizing, nourishing conditioner, like the nourishing conditioning mix. Prevent buildup and mildew by using minimal products and drying hair, before sleeping.

Help! I have seborrheic dermatitis. Can I lock my hair?

Hair can be locked with seborrheic dermatitis. It is important to remain cautious of all products. Natural or synthetic products can cause flare ups. For example, essential oils can trigger flare-ups and irritate the scalp as much as synthetic perfumes or dies can. Wash the locks with a dandruff shampoo to reduce irritation and spritz the hair and scalp frequently with plain Aloe Vera juice, seal with an emollient, such as castor oil. Adding a capful of witch hazel to a liquid shampoo helps immensely for sufferers of an itchy, dry scalp.

Help! My locks are so dry!

If they are dry just SFS: Soften-Feed-Seal! If dry locks are a concern, remember to open up the cuticle by softening the cuticle with the nourishing spritz or purified water. Feed the hair by infusing the nourishing oil into the hair. Then, seal the cuticle with a heavy emollient such as castor oil or the nourishing oil mixture, especially during the winter months. Continue every evening for a week, until the level of moisture desired has been reached. Remember to couple the external moisture with healthy eating and plenty of water intake. Internally, incorporate more healthy foods rich in Omega-3 fatty acids, fiber and nutrients. Eliminate fatty foods that accelerate dandruff and dry hair.

Help! My locks won't hold a curl!

When locks get long, it is harder for them to hold a curl. Consider braid outs or twist out styles that are set with the nourishing gel or just water. Setting the hair while it is saturated with water is best for a tight curl; however, it also takes the longest to dry, plan accordingly. One method for creating hold is known as 'seam welding'. This involves product application down the length of the lock. The process facilitates the formation of physical bonds between adjacent locks with polymer rich ingredients such as Aloe Vera gel, that coats the surface of the locks in the lock, creating clumps of curls via capillary action, which attract the adjacent hair strands to one another. The water will evaporate and the polymers will 'stick' to the lock and hold the pattern until hair is mechanically changed from climate changes or hair alterations. The efficacy of a gel is dependent on climate differences. Assess the climate and

---

[82]See The Holistic Hair Care Chapter.

[83]There are ingredients in some astringents and dish detergents that are on the *Just Say No!* list. Toxins cannot be eliminated 100% from daily use; but toxin exposure can be reduced by being aware!

ingredient. A dry, cold climate will fair well with polyquarternium-11 in the ingredients, because it will infuse moisture into the hair. A good homemade styling spray is 1 ounce of B5 Design Gel by Aubrey Organic mixed with 2 ounces of purified water (mineral water leaves residue) and 1 ounce of organic grain alcohol (vodka). Combine all of these ingredients in a spray bottle, add a couple of drops of favorite essential oil for a healthy hold! When all else fails, set soaking wet locks into braids or onto rollers.

Help! I have loose, stray hairs between my locks and they are everywhere!

If the locks are palm-rolled for maintenance, the hairs will eventually integrate into the lock over time. Minimize movement by always wearing a satin scarf to bed and always cover the head with a satin cap before wearing a hat[84]. If locks are latched for maintenance, be sure to incorporate a 2-step twist technique, which will integrate the stray hairs into the lock overtime. Finger twirling and sealing with a nourishing gel to seal in the loose hairs, is a technique that works nicely for a clean, secure look.

Help! My hair keeps unraveling!

Unraveling routinely happens when lock foundations are started with the wrong method for the hair texture, with coils, or locks started with scab hair. Scab hair is from follicles that have been damaged from years of chemical application or straightening with a petroleum based hair grease. The emerging hair loses its original texture, is usually coarse, and straight. Lock unraveling, also known as slippage, typically happens between months 0-6. To counteract unraveling, be sure to band the hair while washing. Wear hairstyles that involve minimal manipulation. If locks are immature, young, stay away from slippery conditioners and oils, cover the hair with a satin scarf or cap when necessary and stay away from hair coloring during the first year of locking. Consider altering the technique by implementing a 3-step installation method, to prevent unraveling. It will take time, but if the hair is highly textured, it will eventually stop unraveling on its own. Straight hair will require more of an effort to lock. If coils are the installation foundation, wash with the hair net, stocking cap or band to reduce unraveling.

Help! I think I have head lice!

Nine times out of ten, it is not head lice, it's the papilla, the hair root, coming out of the follicle. This is a natural occurrence. Inspect the lock. If there is a hair strand attached to the white bulb, it's naturally shed hair. This is perfectly normal as each hair cycles through the growth stage. The white bulb is released during the telogen phase. The white bulb can be minimized by conventional or unconventional means. Some natural-brewed teas such as chamomile and marigold can lighten the color of the hair, making the bulbs less noticeable. Brewing coffee beans in water and pouring the rinse over the hair, can darken the hair, and lemon juice rinses can lighten the hair as well[85]. An extremely unconventional way to color locks is with a large magic marker. Ink has two big 'Just say No' ingredients: propylene glycol and alcohol. Use judiciously, if at all. Locks can also be brushed with a soft, natural boar head brush to loosen the bulb from the locks. Lock brushing should be avoided on immature locks that are still developing. If locks are older than twenty-four months, brushing them is an alternative. The bulbs will eventually fall off independently, over time. Regular hair dye is an option for some; however, the individual risk/benefit ratio must be considered[86].

---

[84]The Accessory and Hairstyle Chapter

[85]The Holistic Hair Care Chapter

[86]The Holistic Hair Care Chapter

Help! I started my locks with long hair and my friend started locks with short hair. The short locks have grown; but, mine have shrunk. What is going on?

During the first year, the long lock foundation will integrate into the lock transformation process slowly. Any new growth that comes from the scalp becomes integrated into the locking process, meshing methodically with the installed foundation. With long hair, the lock will shrink excessively and not show growth until slowly after the thirteenth month. Around month eighteen to twenty-four months, the lock will finally enter into a noticeable growth spurt. Short hair immediately begins to lock and grow, then all new growth is immediately integrated with the lock foundation, growing and forming into a lock. Long hair takes more time integrate into the lock during the first year, as it transforms from the root-bed and transforms within the installation foundation, then locks will grow. Because this process takes an enormous amount of transformation energy, the process can be painstakingly slow. It's a fact, long hair takes longer to lock; thus, longer to show growth. Ironically, the short and long locks are relatively the same length by year four! Both hair lengths must pay their dues in different ways; however, at the end of the day they miraculously catch up. It's up to the locker to decide the risk/benefit ratio for him /her.

Short-Haired Locker

Long-Haired Locker

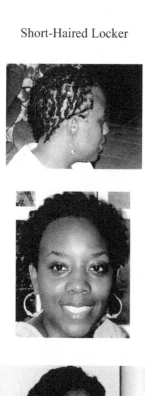
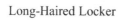
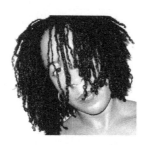

Year One

Year Two

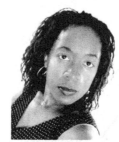
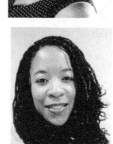
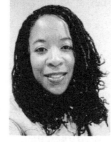

Year Three

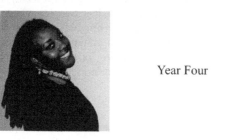

Year Four

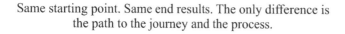

Same starting point. Same end results. The only difference is the path to the journey and the process.

Help! My buds are huge! Will my locks be the size of my bud?

No. Once buds are visible, the locking process has a long way to go. The matrix will begin to intertwine from the bud, extending in opposing directions. Once the matrix is established, the hair will continue to swell and condense, usually thickening to the diameter of the bud. The locks will look much larger than their original installation size. They will begin to tighten into a network of coils and intertwined hair. During the tightening process, the locks will elongate into a uniform lock, and shrink to half their size overtime.

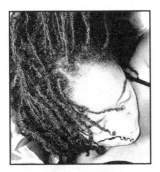

Bumpy locks budding
and condensing

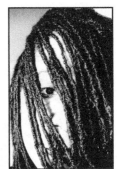

After three years,
locks are
relatively smooth

Help! I have long hair do I have to cut it to grow locks?

No, there are many options available to long and short lockers, there's no need to chop off chemically-free hair that is long. It's important to remain aware of the time and energy for long hair to transform into locks during the first year[87]. Practice good techniques with minimal disturbance and they will lock.

Help! I want to color my locks. Can I color them?

It's safer to color loose natural hair before lock installation. Once locks are installed, within the first 24 months, the hair can unravel. The coloring alters the bonds in the hair, straightening them even more. Even coloring with henna, a natural, protein hair dye, has the ability to straighten the curly bonds in the hair, which can lead to slippage and unraveling. Coloring locks is safest with a trained professional. There are natural rinses to color locks that will turn the locks a different shade over time. Many lockers have lost their locks years after the coloring process, just to learn that the dye left deposits inside of the locks that led to disintegration and hair weakening. If pursuing a color, this is an area where a trained professional is critical. And, not just any trained professional- an individual experienced with locks and coloring is a must!

---

[87]See The Now What Chapter to determine which set of installation locks are for you.

Help! What are these dangling pieces of hair at the end of my locks?

Hair-balls! Hair-balls are simply the shed hair moving down the length of the lock. Some hair-balls will get caught and join in to form the matrix of the lock. The rest will transport to the end of the lock, forming a sealed, rounded end. Others will simply fall when pulled off, the lock will still become a lock; however, the process may result in a coiled, open end that never seals. Some ends will seal, some may not. Locks will even sprout along the shaft of the lock, releasing tiny buds through openings along the lock shaft. A sprout is a hair-ball released along the shaft of the lock and common to free-forming locks.

Help! I need to protect my hair when wearing helmets or hats!

There are satin turbans found most frequently in beauty supply stores. They can also be found periodically at: www.theknottytruth.net. They are similar to the terry cloth turbans worn by Eartha Kitt, but satin. They are perfect for protecting the hair from the damaging friction from hats and helmets.

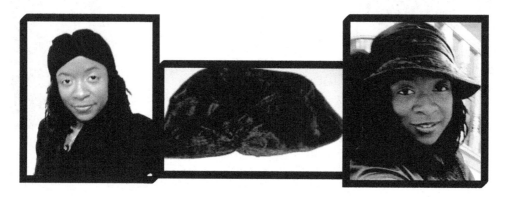

Use a satin cap for protection under hats. Place the cap on the head. Place hat on top of cap and tuck cap away from detection!

Help! I keep getting knots when I latch!

If the knot is in the lock, make sure the lock is pulled all the way through the insertion point. Press down gently on the knot, rolling between the thumb and the index finger, and it will smooth out. Dampen the lock if the knot is stubborn. If a bump forms at the base of the lock, make sure not to tighten the locks all the way to the roots. Stop an eighth of an inch before the scalp. If it's too late, saturate hair with water to loosen the latch. The bump can be at the base of the lock or an actual bump with a white top along the scalp. If the white top manifests, it is the hair-root/papilla and the manipulation must be avoided to prevent permanent damage in the future. Saturate the scalp and hair with water and massage the roots to loosen the hair at the roots, ibuprofen can lessen the pain.

Help! My edges are broken and in a mess from years of damage. Will they grow back in with locks?

Yes! Hair will regenerate amazingly while locking. Highly textured hair prefers to be left alone. When left alone, all types of hair will sprout at the crown, temples and in between locks! Once the scalp gives the signal to the follicles that the trauma from combing, brushing and styling has subsided, the hair will begin to peak out from the follicles and sprout new growth! Spritz daily and seal with an emollient if locks are mature. If they are not mature, sparingly, feed and seal with a light oil such as jojoba. Castor oil is said to contribute to hair regeneration as well, some swear by black castor oil because it's more concentrated and pure, with a strong aroma. To accelerate the process, mix 50:50 with regular organic castor oil.

Help! I wear sun visors but my hair keeps getting snagged by the Velcro! What should I do?

Invest in sun visors that tie in the back. They can be challenging to find-but they are out there! Or invest in a visor with elastic that is covered in the back, for give while protecting your tresses. Periodically, they're listed on www.theknottytruth.net. Another option is to wear the satin cap on top of the hair before putting on the hat, or covering the Velcro with a piece of cloth.

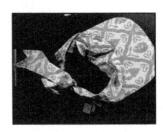

Help! My hair is thinning at the end of my locks. Why is that?

Latched lockers are usually faced with fat ends, upon maturity. The opposite is true for palm-rollers. Palm-rollers may face thinning ends that dangle from years of palm-rolling. This is most noticeable around year two for both sets of locks. The solution is to perform a gentle trim, eliminating the damage. There may be medical causes as well, start here and investigate and never fear snipping the damaged ends while getting to the root of the problem.

Help! There is lint everywhere in my locks. How can I get it out?

•Lint can be brushed out if locks are mature
•Lint can be picked out, however maddening it may be
•Lint can be colored black with a black magic marker[88]
•Lint can be massaged out with a nourishing oil

To massage lint out of locks, with an applicator bottle full of the nourishing oil mixture, squeeze an ample amount of oil into the palm of the hand. Massage the oil into the locks with the thumb and index finger. As the fingers smooth over the locks, the lint will begin rolling onto the fingers. Wipe lent off in a towel and continue. Not only does this remove lint; but, it is great conditioning for the locks! Repeat once a month in the summer-time and biweekly in the winter for nourishment and protection. Try to avoid lent in the first place by:

•Using quality absorbent towels or cotton t-shirts
•Inspecting locks while damp
•Inspecting coats, scarves, clothing for loose strings and balls
•Inspecting hair accessories which are notorious for having lint

If lint still remains, pluck the lent away with a sharp object like a pin.

---

[88]Propylene glycol is inside of ink.

Help! When I wear my hair in a pony tail, my car seat pushes my head forward. What can I do to drive and wear a bun comfortably?

Place a pillow at the lower back, then move the back support of the car seat back. The pillow will provide the cushion and the head rest will not push the head forward. If it is practical, wearing a satin scarf can protect the hair as well, but it won't prevent the pressure on the head forward.

Help! I can pull my locks back in a bun; but, they are not the same length! What can I do to get a full look?

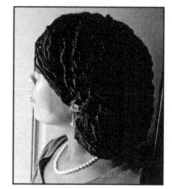

Invest in thin hair nets to complete this look. Pull the locks up with a scrunchie or hair-tie that will secure the locks with flexibility. Place a hair net around the locks in the pony-tail bun. Use hair pins to secure the hair-net. If needed, add synthetic hair to make the bun fuller, cover with the hair net, secure with the pins and use a strand of the synthetic hair around the base of the bun to conceal the scrunchie for an interview ready bun! This technique is very forgiving, giving the appearance of volume for the locked bun.

Help! I am using my creamy conditioner and my locks keep unraveling!

It's important to stay away from slippery oils and creamy conditioners the first year of locking. Change that loose-natural thought process from conditioning and moisturizing to *feeding* the hair (see Index I). By feeding locks nourishing spritzes and rinses, the hair will be fed and nourished and that's adequate! Wait to seal locks with oily emollients (such as black castor oil) after year one when the locks have settled. If not possible, at least wait until the hair has begun to mat to apply a heavy emollient, especially for that ever important SFS process.

Help! My locks are so dry! What should I do?

Remember to SFS: Soften/Feed/Seal locks to seal in much needed moisture, especially during those dry winter months.

Help! My locks are lumpy and bumpy. Is this normal?

Yes, it is perfectly normal for locks to be imperfect, especially the first year! So many new lockers think something is wrong if their locks are not perfectly uniform and smooth. On the contrary, Sisterlocks™ is the only method that comes close to lock uniformity. Other than that, all locks are imperfectly perfect. That's what makes them so stunning. It's better to embrace this quality upfront, rather than obsess over it on the tail end. This hair condition will quickly become a thing of the past if the locker embraces the transformation as the locks, frizz, buds, bunches which are necessary precursors for a lock to mature into a coiled matrix of matted hair.

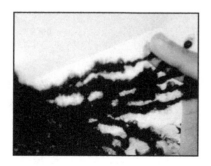

Help! I like to alternate between palm-rolling and latching my locks. Will this impact my lock adversely?

Alternating between palm-rolling and latching could impact lock appearance and health. Alternating between the two methods could lead to the appearance of thick, then thin areas along the lock shaft. The latched section will be smaller than the twisted/palm-rolled section. If lock uniformity is not a big deal, by all means do it. In the future, as the lock tightens and decreases in width, the skinny areas can create stress between the larger areas. Keep a close eye and continue to massage a nourishing oil treatment into the full length of the lock regularly.

Help! I have been doing braid-outs for years and now I see weak areas along my locks. Why?

Too much of anything is a bad thing. It's better to loosely braid or strand twist the locks together for styling. It's important to maintain the proper tension. That would be a loose tension, never overly taught. However, if the damage is already done, STOP! Definitely nourish and evaluate if trimming is necessary. If trimming is necessary, remember to save all cut pieces, they can be sewed back in place with copious care and attention. Locks can also be reinforced with natural extension hair. Wrap the hair around the weakened lock and secure by sewing with a needle and thread.

Help! My locks are flat in the back of my head! What should I do?

This could be from sleeping the same way on the head. Plump up the locks with water and a simple finger twirl to help them form their cylindrical shape. This usually occurs with the older part of the lock. The new growth will grow in correctly and this phenomena will pass as the locks age. Free-formed locks can also grow flat, because they are not palm-rolled or latched for maintenance, as they are left to 'freely' form

Help! I twist my locks and they keep unraveling. Will my hair ever lock?

Even thought twisting is a form of tightening the roots, the true purpose is for a neat, groomed appearance. Highly textured hair will lock and will mat regardless of the twisting/rolling motion. Highly textured hair is porous and coiled in texture. These two traits are absolutely critical for hair to mat and lock naturally. The only exception is straight hair which must be deliberately manipulated in order to lock, because of its protein-rich characteristics and low porosity. So, yes, until the hair mats it will unravel. If it is truly irritating, band while washing or wear styles that keep the twisted formation in place.

Help! Is it normal for locks to be hard and break off?

No! As long as mature locks are cared for via the Soften/Feed/Seal method, at least three to four times a week, the locks will thrive. Locks that are hard and brittle, leading to breakage are malnourished. Stay focused on nourishing mature locks always. Baby to teenager locks can be more challenging to condition. The key with baby locks is to be careful with the feed and seal method. Soften with aloe vera juice or conditioning herbal teas only, massage with a light oil carefully as needed! Immature, rough, scratchy, dry locks can be touched up with an oil from time to time only.

Help! When can I run water through my hair?

As soon as locks are settled, it's safe to rigorously run water through the hair. Once settled, around the teenage stage, it's safe to gently run water through the hair, without fear of unraveling. When locks are palm-rolled for maintenance, it's advisable to wear a hair net or to band the locks into groups of 2-5, to prevent unraveling during the developing baby stage.

Help! I used to be hard headed! Now, that Im locking my scalp is extremely sensitive! What should I do?

Our scalps are stronger when manipulated daily. However, massaging needs to be carefully implemented, to avoid disturbing the locking process. Continue to give the scalp what it needs with daily massages of jojoba oil. Jojoba oil mimics the natural sebum of the scalp and feeds the tender hair follicles, while massages increase blood flow and circulation to the scalp. When circulation is thwarted by decreased manipulation, which leads to decreased blood flow, the scalp will react by becoming 'sore' when touched. This phenomenon is similar to sore muscles that have not been exercised for a long time. Once exercised, the increased activity will lead to irritation and soreness. The scalp is no different and must be exercised to remain strong. Once scalp tissue strengthens, massage jojoba oil into scalp as needed.

Help! I want to use heat on my locks. Is that ok?

No, it's not ok. Keep it simple. If it would burn the skin, it will burn the hair, period. Heat will denature the curly bonds in the hair. Heat will straighten the hair, leading to lock damage and unraveling. Why use heat, when locks can be wet set with water and curlers or braided and twisted? Just say no to heat to curl the hair. If heat is needed to dry the hair, once again, don't! Use a dryer with a cool setting or 'air' setting to help blow the wetness away, coupled with micro-fiber towels.

Help! My hair is not locking as fast as my friend's.

No two heads of hair will lock at the same time. No two heads have the same texture, densities, porosity, length, elasticity or texture. One head of hair does not even have the same biological characteristics throughout the head. So, no two lockers will develop locks the same. No two locker's hair will lock at the same rate. Lock development will be as unique as the individual locker is unique!

Is Nappy Hair Professional?

It took hundreds of years for black women to move from the fields to the kitchen. Then, decades to get out the kitchen and onto blue collar service jobs, now corporate jobs sharing a moniker with our white counterparts. But have black women really arrived post the black love movement of the 1970's? There's damage that reigns in the minds of black women, including myself, who have been taught to perm our hair to get a 'good job.' We've been told to straighten our hair to make other people feel more comfortable with us. Thus, alluding to the fact that our napps are not appropriate for a work environment.

On top of performing twice as well as our counterparts, working long hours and dealing with racism in the workplace, women in the black middle and upper class, or aspiring towards it, have been carefully trained to help other races feel comfortable, beginning with our hair. Because nappy hair texture has been frowned upon by people within the black culture, almost as a right of passage, little girls have been marched to the beauty salon, and conditioned to believe that we are not good enough, and require 'fixing.' As the little girl grows up into a women that brings home the bacon and fries it up in a pan, she has now been conditioned to report to the salon chair almost every month, continuing a lifelong cycle of self-denial and depreciation.

I ask, what is the root of the energy a black woman puts into denying her birth crown of glory?

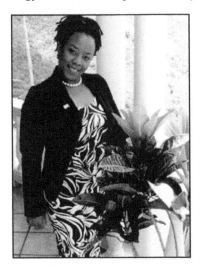

"Nappy hair is professional. The real question is are you?"

PART THREE

PULLING IT ALL TOGETHER

"How will my locks turn out?"

This section references the six core methods of starting locks. Beginning with the most basic of locking methods, organic locks, the reader is taken through the journey of Dilcia and Jordan. They share the simplicity of organic locking, which is, perhaps, the most humble modes of locking. Organic locking requires complete submission to the locking process with little to no intervention. The next journey travels through coils to locks. Considered the most traditional of locks, the journey from coils to locks is shared by Francheska along with Jon, Yvonne and G. George. Backcomb (step 1) locks could easily fit next along the continuum; however, we jump ahead to 2-strand twists locks. Christy shares her journey with help from Natacha, which can be challenging, as this installation method constantly unravels and expands easily. Locking from braids is higher in complexity than 2-strand twists, binding the hair tighter; yet, faced with the challenge of a lingering braid pattern. The advantages and disadvantages of creating beautiful locks on a dime from braids is shared by the author herself, Michele, as she conveys the evolution of locking from braids. Finally, backcomb-interlock combinations are combined into one section. There are four different ways to create locks by back-combing. Brenda shares her locking journey from backcombed-latched-rolled locks, placing her 3-step lock & roll installation right before Sisterlocks. Because the art of backcombing the hair is often interconnected with interlocking, this journey is compiled into this one section, with a breakdown in technique for the traveler who may want a detailed explanation, when jumping off the beaten path. The most complex of all locks are Sisterlocks™, involving a certified installation and maintenance technique. There are traditional locks, that can be cared for by the layman or the professional; and there are Sisterlocks™ which must be installed and maintained by certified consultants or certified clients, making them the most expensive of locks. Shauna and 'Bena share the Sisterlock™ journey: Shauna being a two-year novice and 'Bena a Veteran of five years. By reading this journey and observing the locks, the differences are obvious and the benefits are evident and worth the price for those who choose Sisterlocks™.

When studying the six core lock methods, there is one common theme to notice and that is the end result. No matter how the locks are begun, except for the basic lock formation of organic free-form locks and the complex design of a Sisterlock™, the traditional locks: coils, 2-strand twists, braids and interlocks will typically be indistinguishable from one another at maturity. Organic locks, are still traditional locks, yet will always look uniquely organic. Small to medium Sisterlocks™ usually have distinct appearances as well. Use this section as a guide, keeping in mind that each locker has a unique texture, pattern, density and growth pattern. All of these unique, biological traits influence the look of the mature locks. A unique bouquet of locks evolve on each head of locks; and, the most that any one journey can do is to serve as a 'guide' for the locker. The hair will do the rest. Now, let's look at some fabulous locks on a dime!

CREATING BEAUTIFUL LOCKS ON A DIME!

9

Creating Beautiful Locks on a Dime!
with
Organic/Free-Form Locks

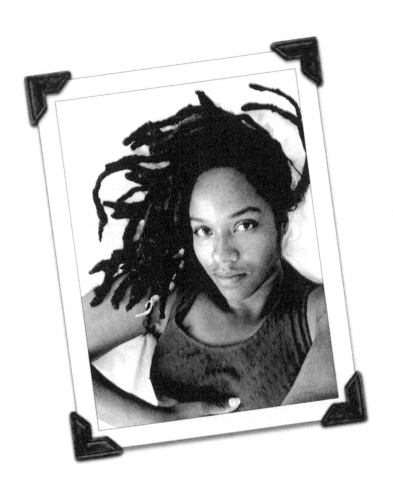

Dreads. Jatta. Ndiagne. Palu. Natty, Ropes, Knots, Organic, free-form locks[88] are all terms referencing an organic explosion of hair that is allowed to grow freely from the roots of the scalp out to the universe. Organic locks are the simplest installation form for locks; and, perhaps the most powerful. Organic locks require a relinquishing of self to a higher power and strength that transcends societal perceptions and self-acceptance. Organic locks represent a lack of concern with the material, symbolizing a relationship to a higher frequency. Some call that frequency their spiritual guide, others Jah, others Bamba, Father, God, Jesus, Shiva, Jatta, others call the name of Haile Selassie, Creator, Jehovah, Vaishnavas, Uhammiri Ogbuide, Anokyi; then, some call them locks: Jah antennae. Organic locks are not about hair, aesthetics or anything that modern society deems as important. Organic locks are about relinquishing self to something higher to gain something greater. Organic locks are the most basic, most humble, most powerful form of locking; and few are called to grow them. But, those who are called take this calling seriously and may look down upon those who choose to journey into lockdom cultivating and controlling their locks along the way. The organic lock is meant to tell the traveler which path to take, not the other way around.

Organic locks can be created on hair that is anywhere from an inch or longer. Starting locks organically is an excellent option for any hair texture with a curl. For Organic Locks, it's especially important to always avoid products with beeswax, shea butter, waxes, detangling shampoo and traditional conditioners, especially when starting locks. It's best to begin organic locks with only water and the appropriate shampoo/soap bar to cleanse[89], accelerating the locking process.

The appearance of organic locks is usually disconcerting to the public who may associate this lock art form with the Rasta of Jamaica. In some African cultures, any form of matted hair is looked upon with disdain and associated with the poor or those who practice witchcraft. From Africa, to America, organic locks can be associated with poverty and filth. An organic locker will continuously have to stand strong and fight this misconception. Organic locks are matted indiscriminately and allowed to grow, without manipulation across the head. If neatness is a concern, many organic lockers wear head scarves and wraps to conceal the hair, keeping the journey sacred and free of negative energy.

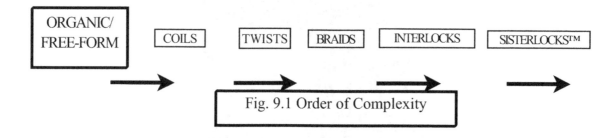

Fig. 9.1 Order of Complexity

Organic locks explode, bud, mat, expand, drop hair-balls, bunch, knot, tangle, and condense. The changes are quite noticeable as the organic locks transform into locks free of boundaries. Organic locks are the simplest lock form; therefore, significantly prone to unraveling! Unraveling is natural and occurs when the hair comes out of its matted formation, and it can continue for months, maybe up to the second year, a unique quality of organic locks. Settling occurs when the hair is left alone, not manipulated and allowed to frizz, knot, tangle and condense without external handling. Settling is an important part of the process during the infancy of the lock foundation, because settling is required for the hair to form the core of the future lock[90]. Because organic locks are not manipulated but allowed to freely form, they frequently capture lint, as nature guides the hair into a random lock formation; resulting in locks of different shapes, forms and sizes.

---

[88]Dreads are usually the preferred name for free-form locks.

[89]A true Rasta or organic free-former may shun the use of any product on the locks, including soap.

[90]See The Lock Evolution Chapter.

Types of Free-Form Locks		
ORGANIC	FREE-FORM	SEMI FREE-FORM
no manipulation	may be a manual install	may be a manual install
no product	may be an organic install	may be an organic install
hair grows free of manipulation from beginning	roots allowed to grow free of manipulation	maintenance is organic with infrequent manual tightenings

Fig. 9.2 Types of free-form locks

Knotty Note

Organic locks: Locks that form freely and are only washed for maintenance.

Free-Form Organic locks: May be installed or organically grown. New growth grows in freely without manipulation.

Semi-Free-Form locks: Locks that may be installed or organically grown and the new growth is manipulated maybe two to three times a year, may or may not be organically maintained.

How to Create True Organic Locks

1. Clean the hair free of residue, it will help the locking process advance.

That's it!

Growing Natural Locks Organically
with
Dilcia

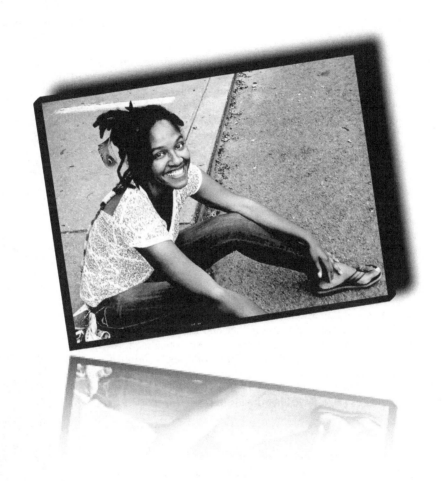

Dilcia's hair texture is loose, bouncy, curly in the Type 2, 3 range. Theoretically, Dilcia's locks would be considered organically free-form and Jordan's locks[92] organic. The difference is in the origin and care of the locks. Jordan's roots are not manipulated, as well as his organic, non-manipulated 'installation'. Dilcia's dreads were installed as 2-strand twists and organically left to form freely without intervention. Even though Dilcia has a straight hair texture with a loose curl in the Type 2-3 range, she is a free spirit, open to letting her hair flow and mature unconstrained. She is not concerned with definition or neatness; and, she allows her hair to pave the way to her journey. As a result, she has unique locks full of character and perfect imperfections that she embraces to the fullest. To keep her locks thrifty and sporty, her only product of choice is lavender oil. Dilcia represents her subset of organically grown locks on a dime well.

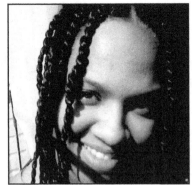

First week of locks

Infant Locks

Extremely confident from the start, Dilcia was able to endure all the crooked glances as her hair napped up in bundles of hair that frizzed, budded and sprouted from her head. The purity of organic free-form dreads is the state of having the will power to let the hair go, along with the audacity to be at peace with the locking process. As her hair knotted up, forming clusters, Dilcia washed her dreads with a natural soap bar and let it be-no conditioners, no oils, nothing but natural soap and water. As her locks took form, they were not neat in appearance; but, artsy eclectic and free to form. Her hair gathered like a tight afro that needed to be picked out, with bee-dee-bee's knotted up at the top, with extreme shrinkage and matting. Many organic lockers, including Dilcia, note extreme shrinkage to only half the original length, within the first trimester! It's difficult for the average woman to free-form, because of hair-length insecurities. Dilcia endured and continued to journey on a healthy path internally and externally. Her locks began to form undefined structures that evolved into the foundation for her mature dreads.

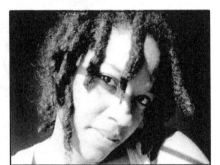

Six month locks

Teenage Locks

After three months, Dilcia was settled into her new-found status as an organic free-former. Her masses of hair continued to group together and mat and clump into undefined dreads. Her straighter hair texture was working to her advantage. Now, defiantly sticking up and growing in many different directions, she continued to watch her dreads sprout. As teenagers, her roots were an undefined mass of afro with the tops sprouting 'branches' of hair. When necessary, scarves and wraps offered some order to her hair as she allowed her dreads to freely form.

Mature Locks

After a year and a half, Dilcia could finally sport a pony tail! That's quite an accomplishment after months of matting and shrinkage and waiting for her hair to show the original installation length. Now, year four, she is still enjoying this stage and continues to embrace her 'natties' as they bloom, elongate and sprout. There's no other lock formation that is simpler and low maintenance, low in complexity with minimal cost, than organic locks on a dime!

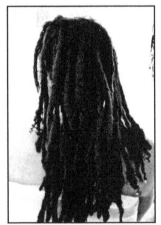

Four-year-old locks

---

[92]The last page of this chapter is Jordan's pictorial journey.

INTERVIEW

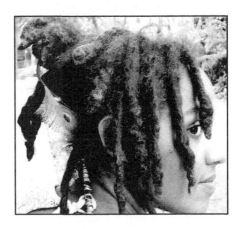

Name: Dilcia Gonzalez (Sole-Rebel)
Maintenance: wash and go, self-maintenance
4-year-old locks

1. Who was the first person you can recall with locks?

    Bobby McFerrin: He taught a master class I attended when I was in junior high school going to Saturday programs at Julliard.

2. Did this person influence you to lock?

    No

3. What did you think of locks before you locked?

    I was mesmerized by them for a little while before I decided to lock. Before then, I never really thought about them, or admire them, really.

4. What do you think of locks now?

    I think locks are the closest thing to what Nature/God/The Creator intended when the human was designed.

5. When you first locked, how did you decide which method would work best for you?

    Through extensive research, and then I stumbled upon *www.nappturality.com*. After that, all the information I needed was in the archives.

6. Who helped you decide?

    No one. This journey has been more internal than external. My mother installed the twists for me, and maintained them for a little bit.

7. <u>What was your physical lifestyle before and after locks and how did that change after you locked?</u>

I'm not sure locks had anything to do with it, so much as they were a result of my change in lifestyle. I was getting quite heavy for my height and for my age, to the point it was starting to affect my health. Before I started my locks, I had gone through a long period of physical neglect-no exercise, bad eating habits, etc.

8. <u>Did you begin living a healthier lifestyle after you locked?</u>

After I locked, I got closer to the Rasta community, and I began eating healthier, and I lost a lot of weight through changing my bad eating habits into good ones, and regular exercise.

9. <u>How has the maintenance routine of your locks impacted by your lifestyle?</u>

Actually, it has freed up so much time! I would spend entire days at the salon getting my hair straightened, even so after going natural, and when I decided not to use the salon to do my hair, I would still have to spend at least 45 minutes detangling my naps. Now it's getting to be work again, as washing longer 'natties' takes longer time in the tub, scrubbing like washing clothes, but I do it less often.

10. <u>Did you choose your maintenance routine because of your lifestyle?</u>

No.

11. <u>How do you feel about skinny locks?</u>

I'm not particularly attracted to them. I feel that they get lost in the distance and look too close to regular hair: I'd rather make a bigger, in-your-face impact. Plus, skinnier locks equals more locks, which equals more work.

12. <u>How do you feel about big, thick locks?</u>

I LOVE thick Locks. They're bolder, and they tend to be more irregular, which to me, is more aesthetically pleasing.

13. <u>How did your feelings about lock size impact your decision to get the lock foundation that you have?</u>

It impacted my decision a great deal. I specifically wanted thick locks, and I always admired Damian Marley's more specifically.

14. <u>How did the size/diameter of your locks change over the years?</u>

It impacted my decision a great deal. I specifically wanted thick locks, and I always admired Damian Marley's more specifically. They started off rather skinny, even though I had the amount of parts I had imagined would be needed to get my desired look. Then, in the teenage stage, they got really poofy and FAT! Then, they condensed a little bit.

15. Did your locks seem to condense and grow skinnier with time or did they stay the same size?

They DID expand and condense, but not that much.

16. If a hairstylist respected your time, was at a convenient location with a good environment would you prefer to go to get your hair done compared to self-maintenance?

No.

17. How much is too much to pay for lock installation of traditional locks (twists, braids, coils)?

Mine were free, so anything is too much. If my mom hadn't decided to help, I still would have installed them myself.

18. How would you describe your personality?

Friendly, afrocentric, nature oriented ? Tricky question.

19. Do you like to do your own hair?

Yes. I'm very touchy about whose hands I let take care of my head in general.

20. How much is too much to pay for lock tightening?

Anything is too much. I would only pay for a style that I cannot do myself.

21. Are your locks heavy?

No, my dreads don't feel heavy at all, except for when they are wet, then I feel the weight.

22. Are your locks the size that you envisioned them to be?

My dreads are EXACTLY what I wanted then to be, but a more detailed version of what I had imagined...I think they're better than what I had hoped for.

23. Is there any advice you would like to share?

Advice: Your hair is happiest in its natural state. Nature knows how to work itself into beautiful things automatically, without our help. That's been my experience. Less is more, and don't worry about they haters, and people who don't understand what's literally going on in and on your head. Don't let your hair run your life, just let it do what it does.

KNOTTY BY NATURE AND ORGANICALLY GROWN WITH TIME[93]

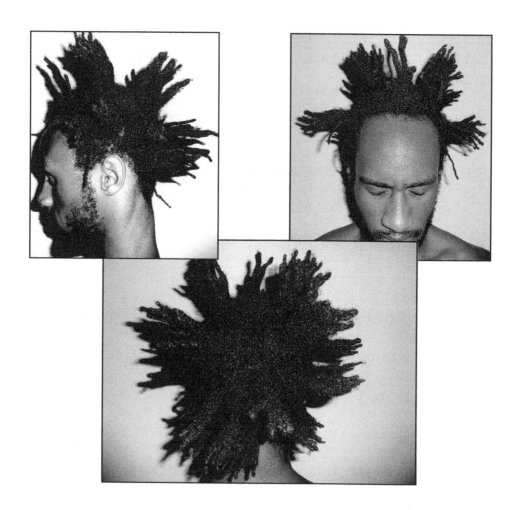

---

[93]Jordan is a world traveler. His locks open doors and attract all kind of people to his journey!

Creating Beautiful Locks on a Dime!

with

Coils!

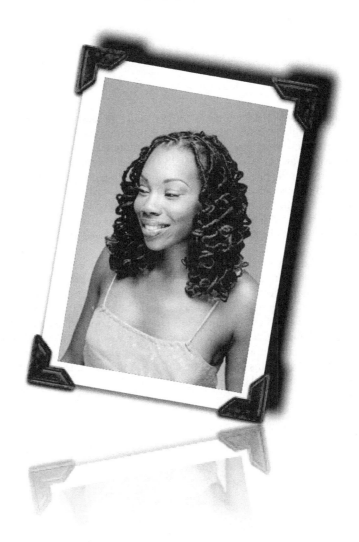

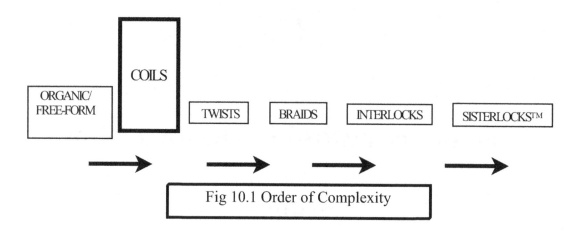

Fig 10.1 Order of Complexity

Coils known also as single strand twists is the traditional way to create locks and are second in order of complexity. Coils can only be installed on highly textured hair, in the Type 4 texture family. Always remember to avoid products with beeswax, shea butter, waxes, detangling cleanser and traditional conditioners, especially when starting locks from comb coils which easily unravel. Coils are usually installed with a gel product, for which the healthy nourishing gel mixture can provide the proper hold and nutrition for the maturing lock. The proper balance must be implemented to prevent an ashy appearance from build up that can occur if too much of the binding agent is applied to the lock. Usually, an amount that covers the tip of an index finger is enough for a one inch parting section. However, the amount must be balanced with the lockers individual hair texture. The denser the hair, more product is required to moisturize. The less dense the hair, the less product may be needed[94].

Even after installation is complete, these locks will unravel until they are settled. Unraveling is natural and occurs when the hair comes out of its lock formation. This is a natural part of the process, with any texture, during the first few weeks of locking. Coils are prone to unraveling! Besides unraveling, coils will also go through a series of changes that include bunching, knotting, tangling and condensing because the lock cannot form until the foundation gets messy, unkempt. Settling occurs when the hair is left alone, not manipulated and allowed to frizz, knot, tangle and condense without external handling. Settling is an important part of the process during the infancy of the lock foundation, because settling is required for the hair to begin to tangle, mesh, intertwine and knot up, forming the core of the future lock[95]. Note that all forms of installing coils look the same. It's wonderful to have options, because there's no right and no wrong way to start them. The key is to just do it!

---

[94]The Holistic Hair Care Chapter

[95]The Lock Evolution Chapter

CREATING BEAUTIFUL LOCKS ON A DIME!

COIL INSTALLATION[96]

0-1 inches: Rubbing

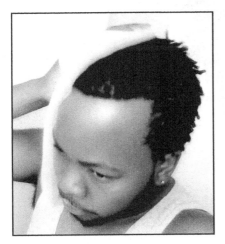

1. Cleanse the hair free of any residue, it will help the locking process advance.
2. On damp hair, apply a small amount of the nourishing healthy hair gel to the head with hands[97].
3. With a luke warm, damp, wash cloth rub towel over the head in circular motions[98].

1-inch and beyond: Comb Coils

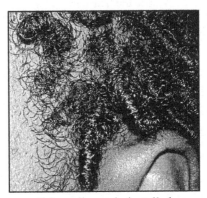

baby coils newly installed

1. Cleanse the hair free of any residue, it will help the locking process advance.
2. On damp hair, section the hair into 1/2" to 1" squares, depending upon the desired lock size.
3. Choose a parting design, such as bricklay, so the locks will lay on top of one another and secure the other hair away from the section with clips[99].
4. Apply a small amount of the nourishing healthy hair gel to the individual section[100].
5. Twist the section around the comb like a spiral and continue to spiral twist the hair with the comb down the full length of the section.
6. Once the coil is in place, put a clip at the root to hold it, repeat and sit under a hooded drier.

---

[96]Now What! Chapter

[97]The Holistic Lock Chapter

[98]We look forward to witnessing John's coil transformation to locks with time, patience and maturity!

[99]The Parts Chapter

[100]The Holistic Lock Chapter

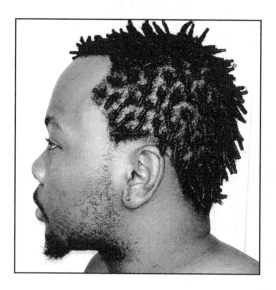

1-inch and beyond: Palm-Roll

1. Cleanse the hair free of any residue, it will help the locking process advance.
2. On damp hair, section the hair into 1/2" to 1" squares, depending upon the desired lock size.
3. Choose a parting design so the locks will lay on top of one another[101] and secure the other hair away from the section with clips.
4. Apply a small amount of the nourishing healthy hair gel to the individual section[102].
5. On damp hair, place the section of hair between the left and right hand between the palms with moderate pressure.
6. Slide the palms in opposite directions, this causes the lock to roll. Be sure to make it roll in the direction that causes the twist to tighten.
7. At the edge of the palm, place the lock at the beginning and repeat the rolling motion.
8. Palm roll each lock for 30 seconds, no longer than a minute.

---

[101]The Parts Chapter

[102]The Holistic Lock Chapter

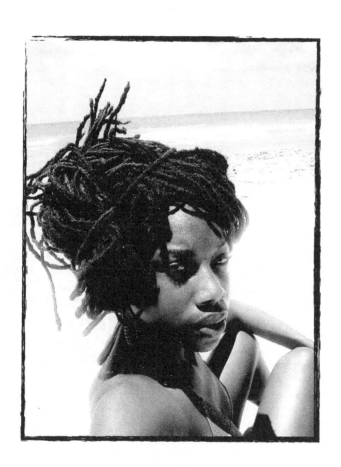

From Coils *to* Locks: Francheska's Journey
with some friends along the way!

Eclectic, fun, energetic, world traveler, model and veteran to the game of locking, Francheska, known by her sistren in the fotki world as the Dread Princess, is known for her stunning five feet or more mane of glory. She's been in the game for a long time and her mane proves the versatility of all locks! Francheska's sense of adventure allowed her to embrace her journey from coils to locks with ease, as she grew deeper spiritually. Francheska's self-awareness awakened and her self-confidence blossomed as her locks transformed from coils to locks. Francheska put vanity aside as she embraced her babies in the early days and her sacrifice paid off with beautiful locks started with the gold-standard of lock installations: coils. Somewhat similar to organic locks, coils require patience. Falling second on the complexity continuum, they are very easy to install; however, they are difficult to care for during the first few weeks of locking. Some with coils sew or pin their coils into bantu knots for months to avoid the naturally occurring pesky unraveling, especially when cleansing the hair. Francheska adorned her head with scarves to keep her locks stabilized, keeping costs low. Fran's favorite products: Moisture: Herb N Life Coconut Hemp, Oyin Handmade Greg's Juice, Olive Oil Shampoo/Conditioner, Dr Bronner's Peppermint soap and Nature's Gate products. When she began locking, picture documentation was not popular, like it is now, so enjoy her journey in words and appreciate the beauty of her seasoned locks, as other's contribute pictorials of the shared journey. They are a testament to the mental and physical growth of growing locks from coils! Locks grown from coils are truly beautiful locks on a dime!

Infant Locks

Francheska, like many who start their locks with coils, found the early days challenging. She didn't know how to wash her coils during the early days, or simply style them. The coils easily unraveled and took a few weeks to begin matting. On top of that, the palm-rolled lock only stayed tight for a week or so. If she sweated or water touched them, they quickly unraveled. To guide her, she solicited the help of her trusty locktician who guided her during those early days, maintaining them with washes and tightening the roots only three to four times per year by palm-rolling. Sometimes a hair net was used to prevent unraveling. Francheska's locks quickly swelled, budded and frizzed as they matted into a matrix that laid the foundation of her beautiful crown today. Her active lifestyle could have interfered with her locking process; but, Francheska prepared herself for the mental aspect of locking from coils by remaining busy, exercising and traveling. Her infamous head wraps protected her tresses on cold or challenging hair days; and, her shower cap prevented her hair from getting wet and unraveling, allowing her hair to transform with minimal manipulation. By week three, the coils were beginning to frizz and appear unkempt. A few times, she touched up her scalp by applying witch hazel to a cotton swab and cleansing the scalp by dabbing it clean. At week four, her hair was washed with the hair net, to minimize unraveling, then her hair was tightened.

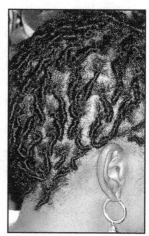

Gilda's Baby Locks

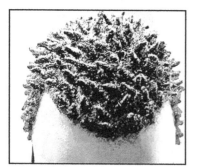

Jon's baby coils on the grow!
Time to tighten!

Teenage Locks

The teenage stage was different than the baby stage; but not better. Good thing Francheska prepared her mind in advance. With head wraps in tote, the teenage stage came, and her locks joined in on the party, sticking every which way defiantly, frizzing, matting, budding and painfully condensing. Francheska's scalp was too tender to pull her locks back, and it became difficult to style the hair, so she let her teenagers spread their wings and fly with scarves, head bands and turbans. By this stage, her locks were matted and did not unravel all the way to the end, just at the root, in between tightenings. She could deal with that. Now, her locks did not unravel easily; and, Francheska was encouraged by the progress! She endured, clinging to the hope that with diligence comes responsibility and a healthy head of locks, as she pressed forward towards maturity.

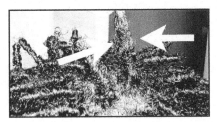

Jon's coils have begun to bud

Mature Locks

When Francheska's locks reached maturity, she was way ahead of the game and setting the bar high for others to follow. Her locks blossomed into a collection of thick locks that crown her well. When she faces challenges from the weight of her locks, she still wraps a scarf to contain her tresses or braids them into a beautiful crown. After ten years of locking, there's not much to do but grow, now. Francheska's locks adorn her crown, cascading down her back and mesmerizing crowds wherever they go. Her wash and go hair has freed her to pursue her passions and enjoy life without being bogged down with the concerns of her hair.

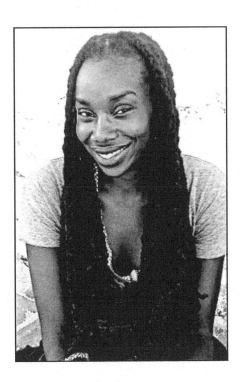

INTERVIEW

Name: Francheska Wilson (Dread Princess)
Type of locks: Coils
Maintenance: palm-roll 3-4 times per year, self-maintenance and professional
12-year-old locks

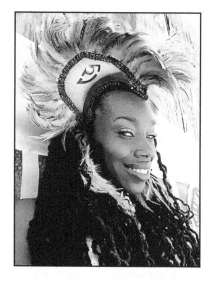

1. <u>Who was the first person you can recall with locks?</u>

My older cousin Zohar. She was a dancer and intellectual. I remember being fascinated with her hair whenever she would visit. I don't think I ever asked her what was going on with her hair. Her hair was like this melting pot of what looked to me like twists and braids. Sometimes I thought it looked really cool and other times I thought it looked messy.

2. <u>Did this person influence you to lock?</u>

I didn't lock until years later but I would say that she had an influence. I knew she wasn't just this artsy, hippie-type woman. The fact that she was very smart and serious about education subconsciously influenced my thoughts about persons with locks. I knew I didn't have to be a "type" to wear locks. I could go to college and be a successful professional with locks.

3. <u>What did you think of locks before you locked?</u>

While beautiful, I thought they would be difficult to maintain and boring because of limited style options. I also thought that you had to have a particular texture of hair to have locks.

4. <u>What do you think of locks now?</u>

They are so flexible and versatile! I've had braids and curls and twists and knots. I've seen locks born of all hair textures. They are easy to maintain and the best thing I've done for my hair.

5. <u>When you first locked, how did you decide which method would work best for you?</u>

My Muslim neighbor had locks and offered to help start me on my journey. When I finally got the courage to BC (big chop), I wasn't aware of the different options for starting locks.

6. <u>Who helped you decide?</u>

The sister who started me on my journey started with palm-rolling and I trusted her completely.

7. <u>What was your physical lifestyle before and after locks and how did that change after you locked?</u>

I was physically active pre-locks but I definitely increased my involvement. Those first few days after getting my relaxer, when my hair was blowing in the wind, water was a no-no. Now, I no longer have concerns about sweating out my 'do. I had a much more carefree attitude about my hair and focused more on enjoying activities like running, dancing and swimming.

8. <u>Did you begin living a healthier lifestyle after you locked?</u>

Yes, I became more cognizant of what I ate by including more fruits and vegetables in my diet. And I spend more time in physical activities. Part of a healthier lifestyle includes feeding the brain and conscious. I increased my involvement in cultural activities and readings.

9. <u>How has the maintenance routine of your locks impacted your lifestyle?</u>

Some people with locks are overly concerned about their neatness. Having an active lifestyle makes me a BIG fan of the wash and go method. I wrap my hair for work and sometimes my hair is wet or conditioned under the material. I am also able to go to the gym during my lunch hour and wrap my hair afterward to go back to work. At this point in my lock journey, it takes such a long time to dry my hair and I don't have the patience to be under a dryer for nearly 2 hours. If I plan to get my hair wet, I usually braid it up and let it dry that way on its own. Or I wash my hair in the gym and sit in the sauna to dry it out. That way, my hair is drying while my body is getting the benefits of the heat. I also LOVE to travel and it really helps being out and about to maintain and style my own hair. I didn't have to worry about finding a hairstylist in Iceland.

10. <u>Did you choose your maintenance routine because of your lifestyle?</u>

Yes, I used to get my hair done by a stylist more often but it became impractical for me and costly.

11. <u>How do you feel about skinny locks?</u>

I feel great about all locks that are healthy.

12. <u>How do you feel about big, thick locks?</u>

I LOVE big, thick locks. These are my personal preference. They have a certain aesthetic appeal that I appreciate.

13. <u>How did your feelings about lock size impact your decision to get the lock foundation that you have?</u>

I didn't really have thoughts about lock size when I first started.

14. <u>How did the size/diameter of your locks change over the years?</u>

I've allowed some of the locks to combine into what I call three-headed dragons where it is one lock at the roots but at the ends you can see that it was originally three locks.

15. <u>Did your locks seem to condense and grow skinnier with time or did they stay the same size?</u>

Both. When I see locks that seem to be getting thinner, I will two strand twist them with an adjacent lock to combine them.

16. <u>If a hairstylist respected your time, was at a convenient location with a good environment would you prefer to go to get your hair done compared to self-maintenance?</u>

I have a great hairstylist that respects my time and has a good location, and a great understanding of locks but I still prefer self-maintenance most of the time because it is easy and you really get to know your hair. If I want something complicated and special then I visit my hairstylist.

17. <u>How much is too much to pay for lock installation of traditional locks(twists, braids, coils)?</u>

That's hard to answer. I think it depends on why you are getting locks and what you expect of them. If this is more of a cultural or spiritual journey for you and you're not concerned about even-sized locks, having your hair "locked" by a pre-determined time or having a particular lock count, then I say call your sisters for help or just get to twisting in your spare moment or if you texture is right, simply stop combing.

18. <u>How would you describe your personality?</u>

Adventurous, creative, assertive, humorous, honest and practical. In other words, human.

19. <u>Do you like to do your own hair?</u>

Yes, absolutely. I've gotten to know my own hair and what I need to do to keep it healthy. I can also see which hair products work best for me and my lifestyle and make changes accordingly. Doing it yourself also enables you to better direct hair professionals when they do your hair. You'll know that some of the locks in the back of your hair have been thinning out so you'll stay away from the tight up-do's for a while. Plus, it's MY hair and I take pride in knowing it better than a paid professional.

20. How much is too much to pay for lock tightening?

Again, I think this depends on your expectations. I do think it is much easier to tighten your own locks than to start them. But not everyone has the time or energy to tighten their locks. I would say that in this day and age, it is much more economical to do it yourself.

21. Are your locks heavy?

My locks are only heavy when they are wet.

22. Are your locks the size you expected them to be?

My locks are the size I envisioned in the beginning.

23. Is there anything you would have done differently that you would like to share?

If I could do it over again, I wouldn't have gotten my hair "done" so much. Early on, I was more concerned about the look of my hair more than its health.

My one piece of advice to a newbie is to get to know your hair. Not only will you save a lot on salon maintenance but you will learn which products work best for your hair.

Yvonne's Picture Journey
from Coils to Locks[103]

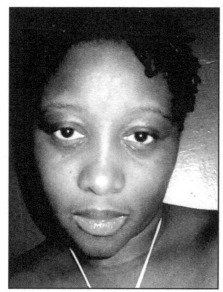

Year 1

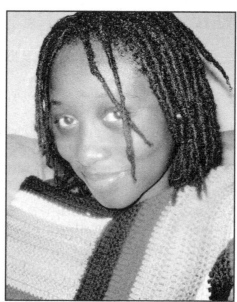

Year 2

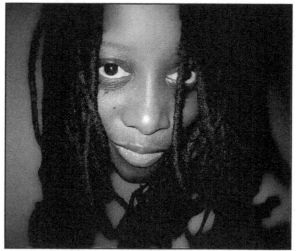

Year 4

---

[103]Extended pictorial transformation from coils to locks shared by Yvonne.

CREATING BEAUTIFUL LOCKS ON A DIME!

G. George's Picture Journey
from Coils to Locks[104]

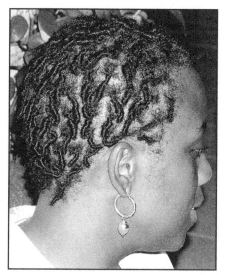

Year 1

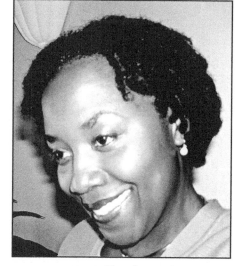

Year 2

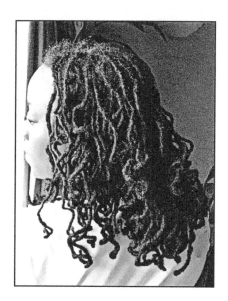

Year 3

---

[104]G. George's pictorial lock journey

11

Creating Beautiful Locks on a Dime!
with
2-Strand Twists!

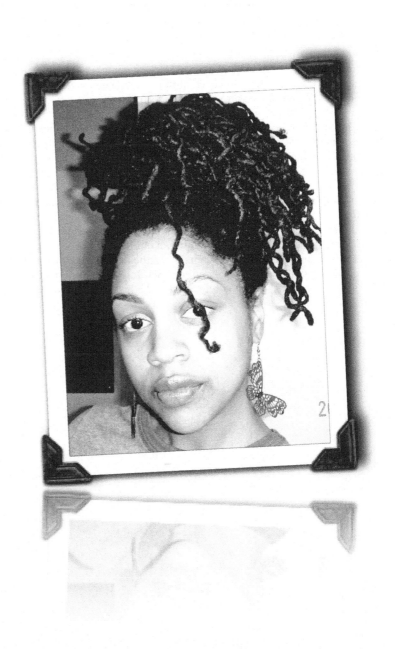

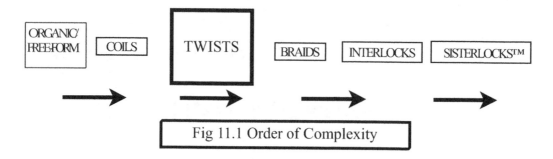

Fig 11.1 Order of Complexity

Two strand twists are also known as double strand twists and they are easy to install. The premise is simple, and can be done on hair that is anywhere from an inch or longer. It is best to only install 2-strand twists on highly textured hair, because they will unravel easily on straight hair. Always remember to avoid products with beeswax, shea butter, waxes, detangling shampoo and traditional conditioners, especially when starting locks from two-strand twists because they can easily unravel. Palm-roll with binders such as mixtures with honey, Aloe Vera gel, or castor oil (such as the nourishing hair gel) to secure the cylindrical lock formation[105]. The proper balance must be implemented to prevent an ashy appearance from build up that can occur if too much of the binding agent is applied to the lock. Usually, an amount that covers the tip of an index finger is enough for a one inch parting section. However, the amount must be balanced with the lockers individual hair texture. The more dense the hair, the more product needed. The less dense the hair, the less product needed.

Even after installation is complete, these locks may unravel until they are settled. Unraveling is natural and occurs when the hair comes out of its lock formation. This is a natural part of the process, with any texture, during the first few weeks of locking. Two-strand twists are prone to unraveling! Besides unraveling, 2-strand twist will also go through a series of changes that include bunching, knotting, tangling and condensing because the lock cannot form until the foundation gets messy, unkempt. Settling occurs when the hair is left alone, not manipulated and allowed to frizz, knot, tangle and condense without external handling. Settling is an important part of the process during the infancy of the lock foundation, because settling is required for the hair to begin to tangle, mesh, intertwine and knot up, forming the core of the future lock[106].

[105]The Holistic Hair Care Chapter

[106]The Lock Evolution Chapter

2-Strand Twist Installation[107]

1. Cleanse locks free of residue, it will help the locking process.
2. On damp hair section the hair into 1/2" to 1" squares, depending upon the desired lock size.
3. Choose a parting design so the dreads will lay on top of one another[108] and secure the other hair away from the section with clips.
4. Apply a small amount of the nourishing healthy hair gel to the individual section[109].
5. Part off the section into two stranded sections.
6. Begin crossing each strand section over the other until the full length of the section is twisted.
7. At the end of the twist, approximately two inches from it, separate the two sections into three sections and braid it to the ends.

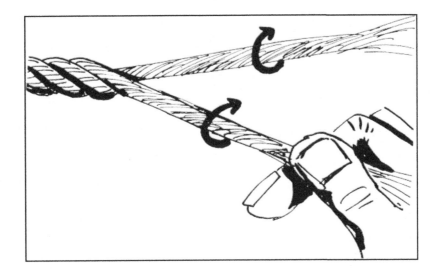

---

[107]The Now What Chapter!

[108]The Parts Chapter

[109]The Holistic Hair Care Chapter

Strung Out
on
Strands!
Christy's Story
with pictorial input From Nat and Michelle

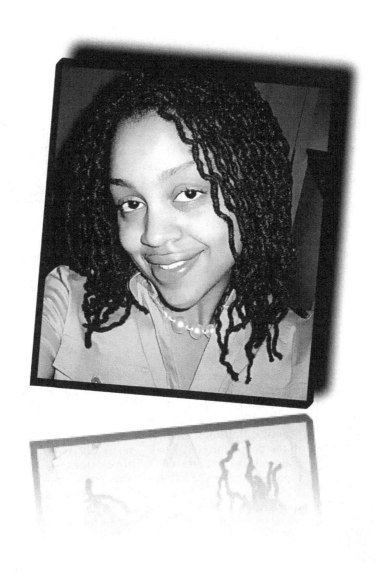

Because two strand twists are among the easiest methods to start locks with, they are quite popular and relatively budget friendly. Two strand twists simply require sectioning the hair, then splitting the section into two parts and wrapping the two parts around one another, securing the ends. For Type 4 hair, two strand twists will begin to lock quickly, losing its initial texture design, unraveling into undefined locks quickly in the first few weeks. Twists allow lockers like Christi to progress quickly, because twists are weaved around only two sections of hair. As a result, the pattern will quickly fade away as the locking process matures quickly. Twists can be installed at any size, from micros to large and maintained by any method: palm-rolling, latching or free-forming. Christi was excited to have locks that she could maintain financially as a struggling college student. The greatest expense was the cost of her preferred styling products that she replaces maybe twice a year: pure Coconut Oil, Extra Virgin Olive Oil and Parnevu Tea Tree Shampoo and Conditioner. Now, that's fabulous locks on a dime!

Infant Locks

Christy grew her locks quickly, after transitioning and wearing her loose natural hair for over a year. Like a lot of lockers, Christy had a false start as the bumpy road to lockdom began. Her initial installation was comb coils installed by a locktician. After enduring weeks of an itchy scalp, she felt empowered to re-start her journey with 2-strand twists, installed by her room-mate. Now, seven years later, she has over two feet of lovely medium sized locks maintained by palm-rolling. The huge obstacle she faced during the early days was unraveling. The 2-strand twists quickly unraveled many times during the first few weeks as the hair quickly transformed into locks, frizzing, shrinking and budding. Then, the hair began to mat and lock around week twelve. Once her hair began to mat, Christy chose to move forward with the two strands intact. When washing her hair, she was careful and keep her hair nourished with water. If her scalp was extremely itchy, she would massage some jojoba oil lightly into the scalp to sooth and nourish the scalp and hair.

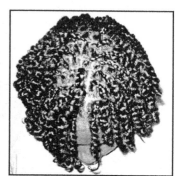

Michelle's 2-strand twists

Teenage Locks

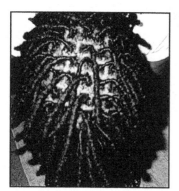

Teenagers! Month 5

Because of the unraveling, Christy dealt with condensing, swelling, frizzing, thickening of her locks, during the teenage stage. Two strand twists worked well for Christy as a college freshman. Having attended an HBCU, she was in a supportive environment in the Mecca of locked beauties: Baltimore, MD. She saw naturals with baby locks at school and in the community on a daily basis. Christy also saw locked lovelies with mature locks that grazed their back sides, swaying in the wind. With this type of supportive climate, she knew that patience would produce a flowing garden of locks on her head as well. Her locks formed a strong foundation that anchors her mature locks today. For a college student on a budget, 2-Strand locks were a perfect start to a hair-drama-free college life.

Mature Locks

Christy's locks are seven years old and quite mature. Her locks have tightened and are now compact, thinner. She continues to palm-roll her lovely locks every 4-6 weeks herself; but, no longer worries about unraveling. Frizz is at a minimum and post-wash braidouts complement her crown, minimizing any post wash root frizz. Her challenges now: How to style her hair and shorten her shampoo-drying times, while accommodating her long, compact locks that retain water.

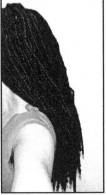

7-year-old locks

INTERVIEW

Name: Christy Skipper (Karamel)
Type of locks: 2-Strand Twists
Maintenance: palm-roll, self-maintenance every 4-6 weeks
7-year-old locks

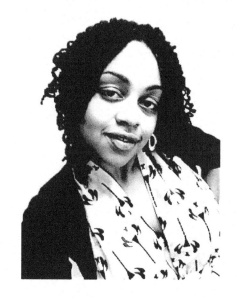

1. Who was the first person you can recall with locks?

    Shaza from A Different World played by Gary Dourdan.

2. Did this person influence you to lock?

    No, but he was easy on the eyes.

3. What did you think of locks before you locked?

    I don't remember thinking much about locks before I locked. I would imagine that I thought that they were impossible for me to grow and a style that I'd never consider. Oh, how things change!

4. What do you think of locks now?

    I think locks are beautiful, unique, big small, colorful, tangled, amazing works!

5. <u>When you first locked, how did you decide which method would work best for you?</u>

I first locked by accident. I'd been relaxer free for over a year and decided to do the big chop. My stylist initially used gel twists to achieve an off the face, light and easy to maintain style. When I went back for a second visit she mentioned that I could grow locks from the gel twist style. She re-styled into gel twists and I went on my way…a week or two later the itching became unbearable and I washed them out. Fall semester began and a friend of mine two-strand twisted my hair with a combination of grease and oil. My scalp wasn't irritated, my hair had grown a little and the two-strand style was really pretty and easy to sleep on. I never washed them out and hence my locks were born….

6. <u>Who helped you decide?</u>

No one helped me decide which way would work best for me. I knew what didn't work (gel twists) and I really liked the two-strand style… it sort of just happened. I will say that attending an HBCU in Maryland really exposed me to locks and inspired me to keep my two-strands in. In my opinion, Baltimore is Lock City. They're everywhere!

7. <u>What was your physical lifestyle before and after locks and how did that change after you locked?</u>

Before my big chop I actually had had a doctors visit a few months before and learned that I had high triglyceride levels …I was only 21!!!! I loved fast food and anything fried. I never exercised…and I was a victim of the freshman 15 and the sophomore 15 more…

8. <u>Did you begin living a healthier lifestyle after you locked?</u>

My healthier lifestyle actually began a few months before my big chop. After learning about my high triglycerides I tried a vegetarian diet (that lasted about 3 weeks) and began exercising. I dropped close to 30 pounds and have managed to keep it off 6 years later… for the past 5 years or so I've been very good about exercise and maintaining my weight. January 2009, I began a meat free diet and plan to continue that for as long as possible.

9. <u>Has the lock maintenance routine impacted by your lifestyle?</u>

Although I work out four to five days a week, I do not wash and re-twist my locks any more than usual. I tidy up the edges and slick back into a pony tail to give it a neat appearance but other than that I still stick to a four to six week re-tightening timeframe.

10. <u>Did you choose your maintenance routine because of your lifestyle?</u>

I chose my maintenance routine because I think the less I have to manipulate my hair the better off it will be.

11. <u>How do you feel about skinny locks?</u>

I have skinny/slim locks and I have my days where I love their size and other times I think about combining… A lot of times people confuse my locks for braids.

12. <u>How do you feel about big, thick locks?</u>

Big locks are gorgeous and I'd love to combine. I feel like bigger locks would take less time to wash and maintain. Also I feel that some of my family members wouldn't want me to get bigger locks… I know this for a fact. My mom, sister and aunt do not want me to combine. Their opinions (surrounding my hair) influence me greatly…so until I become stronger and more secure with that decision I'll keep my locks thin.

13. <u>How did your feelings about lock size impact your decision to get the lock foundation that you have?</u>

I had no knowledge of lock size at the time I began my journey. From the size of the two strand twists I knew I'd have a lot of locks…I feel like they were a bit larger before they started to compress and coil and mat together.

14. <u>How did the size/diameter of your locks change over the years?</u>

Again, I feel like my locks compressed together more and more after the first year and a half, two years. Some of my locks are the size of sharpie…some are thinner than a number 2 pencil.

15. <u>Did your locks seem to condense and grow skinnier with time or did they stay the same size?</u>

Yes my locks seemed to condense and get skinnier. I don't expect them to get any thinner with time (crossing my fingers).

16. <u>If a hairstylist respected your time, was at a convenient location with a good environment would you prefer to go to get your hair done compared to self-maintenance?</u>

I would still do it myself. Maybe I'd visit the stylist for up-dos or deep conditions but regular maintenance would be my job. Although there are advantages to having someone else doing your hair (i.e. not having to do it yourself!), I dislike paying someone for something I can do myself.

17. <u>How much is too much to pay for lock installation of traditional locks (twists, braids, coils)?</u>

More than $80.00 is way too much. When I look at pricing guides for start locks or however you name it, I get turned off. "Installing" locks doesn't require any special chemicals so I don't understand why the fees are so high. It's a definite turn off for those interested in achieving this style.

18. How would you describe your personality?

Introverted, a bit anti social, quiet, would rather listen than talk, watch rather than interact…. I am also very goofy and silly but it takes awhile to become comfortable enough to show this side to others.

19. Do you like to do your own hair?

I don't LIKE to do it but I like that I don't have to depend on anyone else to do it. I love the end result but the time it takes to do it is a bit of a downer!

20. How much is too much to pay for lock tightening?

When I used to have my hair maintained by a stylist in '04 and '05 I was used to paying $40-$50 tops! I still think that's the most reasonable price…anything beyond that is ridiculous.

21. Are your locks heavy?

My locks are only heavy when they're wet. When dry, they're manageable unless I put them in a ponytail. In that style I do feel the weight of them; but, it's not unbearable.

22. Are your locks the size you envisioned in the beginning?

I wasn't sure what size locks I'd have or even what they would look like. I was fascinated though at how they compressed and became thin as they locked up. As I mentioned before I'd love to have really thick locks but am nervous about the transition process.

23. Is there anything you would have done differently (one piece of advice to give a new locker)?

Definitely! I would have used a satin bonnet and pillow case religiously in the beginning to help combat lint and to maintain moisture. I also would have moisturized my hair on a regular basis.

Transforming Pictures of Nat's Beautiful Large 2-Stranded Twists to Locks[110]!

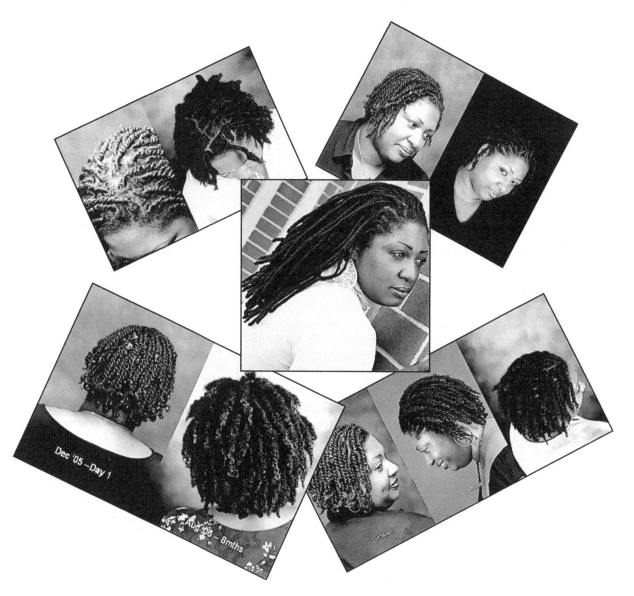

---

[110]Diva alert! Nat's transforming pictures of the transformation process from 2-strand twists to locks!

CREATING BEAUTIFUL LOCKS ON A DIME!

Creating Beautiful Locks on a Dime
with
Braids!

12

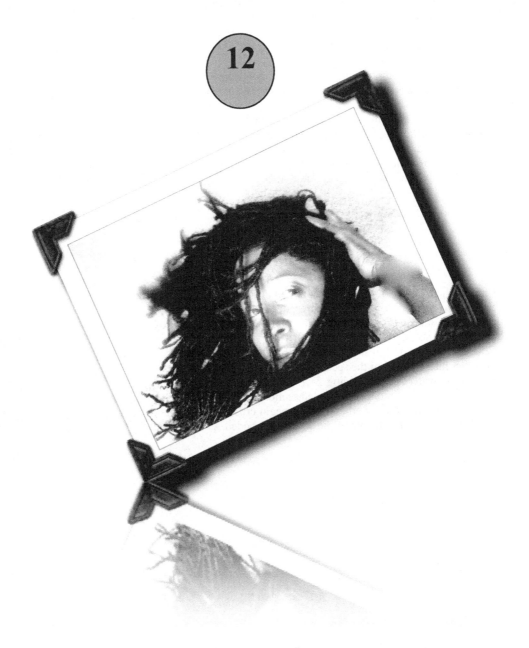

Braids are simple, and can be done on hair that is anywhere from an inch or longer. Starting locks from braids is an excellent option for any hair texture with a curl. Even though braids are relatively secure, it's good to always avoid products with beeswax, shea butter, waxes, detangling shampoo and traditional conditioners, especially when starting locks. It's best to begin braids, like most locks, with only water to accelerate the locking process, waiting to introduce conditioners once the locks have matted.

The appearance of braidlocks can be controlled by the tension of the braid lattice. Braids can be installed with a loose lattice or a tight lattice. If braids are installed with a loose lattice, they will swell quickly, lose the braid pattern quickly and expand. If braids are installed tightly, they may retain their braid pattern for a considerable amount of time, lasting up to four years, it will depend upon the hair texture pattern. A tight braid pattern also resists locking versus the loose braid lattice. There are advantages to both. If neatness is a concern, a tight braid lattice will look like braids for a longer amount of time; however, a loose lock pattern will transform to locks almost immediately. If the locker is anxious to begin the locking process, a loose lock lattice could begin to transform within the first trimester of locking.

Even after installation is complete, the braidlocks may unravel until they are settled. Unraveling is natural and occurs when the hair comes out of its lock formation. This is a natural part of the process, with any texture, during the first few weeks of locking. Because braids are one step up in complexity from 2-strand twists, they are slightly prone to unraveling; however, not as much as 2-strand twists, coils and organic locks. As a result, braids will also go through a series of noticeable changes that include bunching, knotting, tangling and condensing. Settling occurs when the hair is left alone, not manipulated and allowed to frizz, knot, tangle and condense without external handling. Settling is an important part of the process during the infancy of the lock foundation, because settling is required for the hair to form the core of the future lock[111].

Braid Installation[112]

1. Cleanse the hair free of residue, it will help the locking process advance.
2. Section the hair into 1/4" to 1" squares, depending upon the desired lock size. If uncertain, start with microlock 1/4" partings and combine over time until desired lock size is attained.
3. Choose a parting design so the locks will lie on top of one another[113] and secure the other hair away from the section with clips.
4. Spritz with water before braiding.
5. Part off the section into three stranded sections.
6. Using an underhand or overhand stitch, begin crossing each strand section over the other until the full length of the section is braided.
7. Braid to the end or leave only 1/4 loose[114].

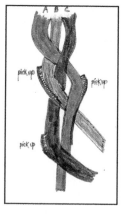

---

[111] The Lock Evolution Chapter

[112] The Root of the Matter Chapter

[113] The Part Chapter

[114] The more braid that is left loose, there's a greater probability for thickening, bunching and variability. If a tight, uniform lock is desired, braid tightly, all the way to the end of the braid.

Tied up
in
Braids!
Michele, The Author

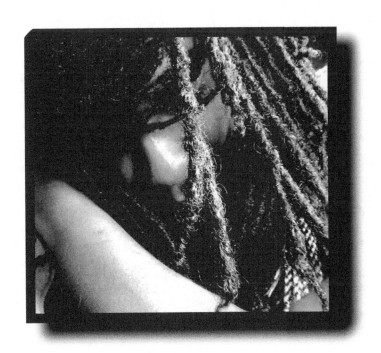

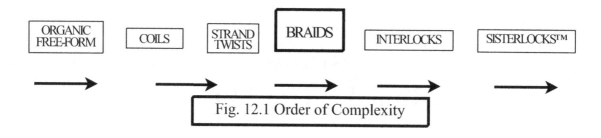

Fig. 12.1 Order of Complexity

Yes, braids can create beautiful locks too! Not too long ago there was a theory that locks could not start from braids. That theory has been dispelled by some of the original pioneers that have created beautiful locks from braids such as Alice Walker's, now gone, dynamic, thick, juicy palm-rolled locks which are on display in the book Dreads[115]. Closer to home, there were sisters on the internet that encouraged me with their beautiful locks. There are e-books on the topic, blogs and online communities. Some call them braidlocks, others bradelocz. I call mine microbraidlocks that transformed to braidlocks that transformed into locks. However, the only difference is size and name preference. After researching, asking questions, studying online picture albums, I printed off pictures from the internet and set off to find someone to braid my hair in 2006. I was told by a locktician that it was not possible to grow locks from braids, she insisted I had to get Sisterlocks™. Since I had the pictures, I commenced to install my own braids. I would have paid her to do it; however, she said it couldn't be done. With my Type A personality, that's all I needed to hear, to prove that theory wrong, doing it myself!

I chose braids because I worked in a super conservative industry. I needed an installment foundation that would keep my hair under the radar and neat. I put 400 starter micro-braids in my hair, forfeiting my deposit on the starter Sisterlocks™. After much research and hesitancy about the price, I knew that she preferred to maintain control of her journey; but, I needed the flexibility to self-maintain, because of my long natural hair length. The Sisterlock™ price was equivalent to my house payment, and that wasn't going to happen. After fourteen hours, my microbraids were installed and five years later, I have locks. I maintain a low budget on hair care products by stocking up on real African Black Soap, Aloe Vera juice, and gel, essential oils, castor and olive oil for moist, soft locks.

[115]Pagano, Francesco (Author); and Alfonse (Joint Author); Walker. Dreads [DREADS -OS]. Grand Rapids: Artisan Publishers, 1999. Print.

Infant Locks

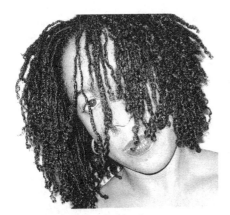

The Beginning

My baby locks started as neat, little braids that danced around my face in spring coils and curls that surprised me. As a loose natural, I preferred two strand twists, not braids. The beauty of the braids surprised me. There were so many questions and worries as I worried about issues like parts and lock size and frizz. By week three, the frizz took over my head and my hair shrunk to less than half of its length. In the back, the braids were unraveling, bunching, slipping, sealing and flaking from the excessive petroleum-based locking gel used to install the braidlocks. I learned that was a big no, no and frequent shampoos with ACV rinses eliminated the gel, and accelerated the lock formation process. Eventually, I learned that banding helped reduce bunching and slipping when I cleansed my locks. Because of the excessive unraveling, it took more time; but it worked. As a result, I now just suggest that locks are installed on clean damp hair only. The front braids were braided into a tight lattice because of the straighter texture; however, retained their pattern longer because of the tight lattice. Needing to keep a neat appearance, I didn't want my braids to unravel and swell. I was less meticulous about the back and experimented with looser braid lattices and open ends, because of my tight texture in this section of my head. Braid-outs became my favorite style to counter frizz.

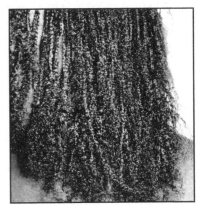

Baby microbraidlocks on A.Karim

Teenage Locks

It seems like overnight my soft, spongy, curly braids disappeared, replaced with hard, undefined sections of matted hair. These teenagers weren't cute like the curly braids, they were part braid and part hardened lock, they misbehaved and stuck up in weird places and curled in unexpected places. I began combining locks that expanded, needing more support at the roots. The braidlocks also began to bunch and bud, making the individual lock appear quite ugly-but collectively beautiful and different, as hair-balls began to dangle from the ends of my locks. I caught strangers giving me the side-eye as if wondering when I was going to do something with my hair. My conservative father patted my head like a Chia Pet and co-workers asked me if liked my hair 'like that.' Supportive websites became my support network: www.nappturality.com, www.fotki.com and www.blogspot.com. Mentally, this journey was taking me to unchartered territory; and, for the first time, I began to embrace myself in spite of my hair. The epiphany fueled me forward.

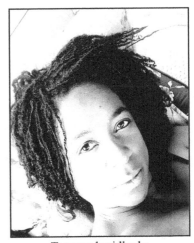

Teenage braidlocks

Mature Locks

Now, accepting my locks even more, month twelve I combined more locks. My locks began maturing and peaked at month fourteen. I always enjoyed taking pictures of this journey because pictures always show a different story than the naked eye can see. By month fourteen, for the first time, I could see locks in the pictures, unlike real life. My locks had a long way to go, but more than half of the former braid was now a lock from the root down. I couldn't believe that all those tiny knots I made in my new-growth lead to a cylindrical lock! Because the thick braids at the ends of some of my locks bothered me, I decided to unravel more of the stubborn braids that remained at the end of many braidlocks, a move I would later regret[116]. At month eighteen, my locks were finally, once again, the length that they were when installed and visibly growing! The thick locks that were combined months earlier now condensed even more as the combined lock section started the locking process over again. It was not until year three that the braidlocks began to tighten back to their original size. As the portion of the locks tightened, the former braid became a nub of its former twelve inch glory. Now, at the ends, the twelve inch braid began to clump into a 1-1.5 inch mass of hair. The locks that were unraveled to eliminate the braid were wide, bulky and noticeably larger than my lock shaft. The combined locks became branches of a tree that gave fullness and volume to my locks. At my four year lockaversary, my locks of hair grew to bra strap length for the first time in life. Now, with my locks in a continual growth phase-the nubby braids were cut off; and, my lock journey began again, this time without any braids.

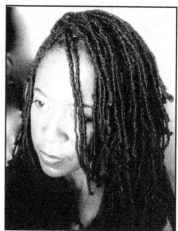

Year 4! No more braids!

---

[116]The more braid that is left loose, there's a greater probability for bunching and variability. If a tight, uniform lock is desired, braid tightly, all the way to the end of the braid, as much as possible.

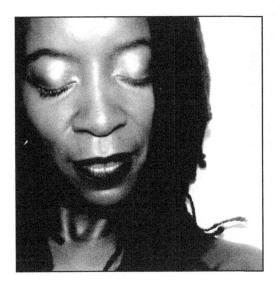

INTERVIEW

Name: Michele George (Cheleski/Shell-skee)
Type of locks: Microbraidlocks
Maintenance: 4-6 weeks self-maintenance/4-point reverse interlock(latching) rotation with 2.5 inch hair-pin
4-year-old locks

1. <u>Who was the first person you can recall with locks?</u>

Probably my cousin, Joy. She was the first person in my family with locks. Watching her locks mature, was the first time I became impressed with locks. Before that time, my perceptions were all off. But, it was when my cousin Jason, her brother, locked his hair that I was sold.

2. <u>Did this person influence you to lock?</u>

He exuded a confidence that spoke to me. After months of researching different techniques, as soon as I returned from the family gathering, I locked my hair down immediately!

3. <u>What did you think of locks before you locked?</u>

I was not impressed. I just did not physically or mentally identify with locks. Most locks I saw were free-form locks and I did not get that, then. I did not get a lot of things! But, as my growth matured, my vision expanded and I began to see and draw upon the beauty of all locks with that maturity.

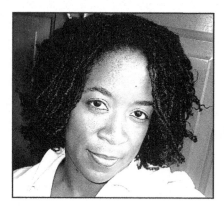

4. What do you think of locks now?

Well, locking for me is personal. I locked out of a necessity to preserve my hair. I never thought that I would lock. It was not an aspiration for me. I locked because of the nightmare I experienced week after week as I washed and styled my hair for 72 hours straight. The planning, products and manipulation were exhausting. That necessity has transformed into a beautiful journey as I've learned to embrace my God-given beauty and see that beauty even when I'm not looking physically beautiful. It's been a deep, transcending evolution for me. However, I don't feel it's such a deep spiritual journey for everyone. So, I have learned not to assign that mantle to all with locks. People are people, thus assumptions are dangerous to make even amongst lockers, as many will lock for the pure aesthetics of it and get rid of them the next day. So, I've learned that my journey is personal, it's best to keep it that way.

5. When you first locked, how did you decide which method would work best for you?

Because of the length of my hair, it boiled down to two methods: Sisterlocks™ or Braidlocks. I needed a method that could avoid detection, remain neat and manicured for my length of hair and organic, coils and 2-strand twists were not secure enough for my lifestyle. I worked in an industry where locks were unheard of for African American women, while braids were acceptable. After an initial Sisterlock™ consultation resulted in a price quote of $900.00 for installation and $3-400.00 for tightenings every 4-6 weeks, I went with micro-braids. A sister in my Fotki album family by the name of A. Karim had fine, microbraidlocks that she started on her own. It clicked to me that I could do the same and maintain the roots in a rotation similar to Sisterlocks™ and have the look that I want as well.

6. Who helped you decide?

The Sisterlock™ consultant!

7. What was your physical lifestyle before and after locks and how did that change after you locked?

I became a Certified Personal Fitness Trainer in 2003. After three to four years of healthy living and transitioning due to hairdresser problems, money etc. it clicked. I began researching everything I put in and on my body. When I learned that chemical relaxers were made of the same ingredients as Liquid Drano, I was enraged and went natural. Now, I'm even more physical, in my 40's. I take two to three hour long bike rides with my husband on the weekends, I exercise even more and I even submersed my whole body and head in the ocean for the first time this summer in the Gulf! I was laughing and crying the same time, because I could feel my locks floating in the water and embracing all of me. I haven't felt that since I was a carefree child jumping in the pool before mommy could catch me and put that swim cap on my head. I was free and locked! I'm so excited about all the other adventures that I

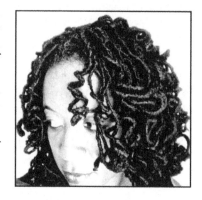

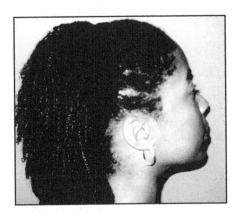

can enjoy now that I have wash and go hair!

8. Did you begin living a healthier lifestyle after you locked?

My healthy lifestyle has evolved even higher. I eat a diet of God-made/ Man-made which focuses on eating foods that God made. If I can't pronounce the ingredients, I try not to eat it. I also practice two or three meat free days a week. I see the difference in my skin, hair and overall health. My goal is to one day become a Vegan, probably when my kids are grown.

9.How has the maintenance routine of your locks impacted by your lifestyle?

I incorporate lock maintenance into my life. I have hair-pins all over my house, car, purse and I'll latch a loose root anywhere! So, there's no stopping me! I also enjoy doing it. It soothes me and I enjoy my daily head massages, as well. That's about the most maintenance that I do!

10. Did you choose your maintenance routine because of your lifestyle?

Yes! I have an active lifestyle as a working mom of two boys and exerciser. I began to resent my hair when it was natural and loose and I did not want that adversarial relationship with my locked hair. Latching the roots myself is the best thing for my Type A personality, because I could never imagine going through the bother of tightening my roots, and watching them unravel when palm-rolled. To me, what's the point? But I respect others that choose to do so.

11. How do you feel about skinny locks?

That's all I used to want. With maturity my vision of beautiful locks has evolved. I've even enjoyed combining locks over three to four times, to increase their size. I now see the beauty in all locks and I think options are great.

12. How do you feel about big, thick locks?

I see the beauty in all locks and I think they are great.

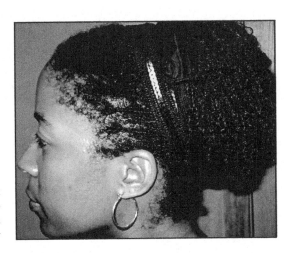

13. How did your feelings about lock size impact your decision to get the lock foundation that you have?

In the beginning I wanted skinny Sisterlocks™ that looked like strands of hair. Even though I did not keep them small, I'm glad I started with micro-braids because I've been able to re-create my look many times, combining them and watching the locking process evolve again and again.

14. How did the size/diameter of your locks change over the years?

My idea of size has grown over the years, I think the best size is what works for the locker, because that's who has to deal with it day in and day out, not me. At first my locks were skinny braids, then they expanded two to four times their width, now, they've condensed down to almost their original size, amazing.

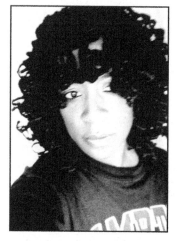

15. Did your locks seem to condense and grow skinnier with time or did they stay the same size?

They condensed, getting shorter, tighter, wider year one through the end of the year two. At year three, they began to condense, tighten, growing skinnier, compact and longer. I would say, during year five, of locking, my locks are now about the same size as installation, even though the root-bed is significantly larger now. This process is amazing to me!

16. If a hairstylist respected your time, was at a convenient location with a good environment would you prefer to go to get your hair done compared self-maintenance?

I would always prefer to do my hair myself. I have so many idiosyncrasies and I'm so picky that I would annoy myself annoying someone doing my hair. I know each and every lock intimately. I know what it needs and how it needs to be treated. I'm very particular about products that are put in my hair as well. But I must say, there is room for me to be flexible as I age. Just not now!

17. How much is too much to pay for lock installation of traditional locks (twists, braids, coils)?

A reasonable price is a maximum of $60.00 for twists or coil installation and approximately $125.00 for braids in the midwest.

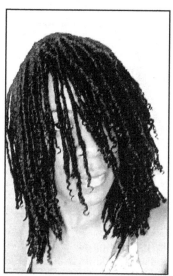

18. How would you describe your personality?

Im definitely Type A. I prefer to be in control. I'm very independent and inquisitive. Im a trained researcher and I apply that to every aspect of my life.

19. Do you like to do your own hair?

Love. It!

20. How much is too much to pay for lock tightening.

Tightening traditional locks should only take no more than $75.00 in the midwest. I do it for free for my own locks.

21. Are your locks heavy?

No, my locks are not heavy at all.

22. Are your locks the size that you envisioned them to be?

Sure, I wanted locks and was willing to take the journey with the end in mind. Five years later, Yes, Im pleased. Besides raising children, it's the most self-sacrificing journey I've taken that required me to relinquish my desire to control situations, let go and let be and I continue to learn a lot about myself because of it.

23. Is there anything you would have done differently your first year of locking, looking back?

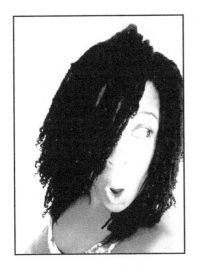

I encourage women to seek the encouragement of someone who has locked their hair recently through online pictures albums, YouTube videos or real life. However, it's important to remain balanced. It's so easy to develop lock envy: the state of lusting over someone else's locks. Just like no two heads of hair are the same in texture, shape and size, no set of locks will be identical to another's. For example, Sisterlocks™ is the most uniform system on locking out there today; however, a small set of Sisterlocks™ is not going to look the same on me as on another sister. My texture, density, porosity is different than another's and my small locks may swell up and another's may remain thread-like skinny. The beauty in locks is embracing the simplicity of their design, respecting the unique transformation process and accepting the perfection in the imperfections.

Another major concern lockers have with braids is the pattern. The pattern never bothered me. Because of my employment situation in corporate world, I wanted my hair to have the appearance of braids as long as possible. For me, that lasted until month 13. Many employment policies are friendly to braids, not locks. As a result, I was fine with my decision. Because the new growth is what actually becomes the lock, the braid was at the tip of my lock by year three. Once again, it was not noticeable unless you stared at my hair and it was only on a few of my locks that I braided with very tight lattices and a straight hair texture. By year four, those old braids were bulky and unappealing, so I snipped them away anyway. I would begin my locks with braids in a heart beat.

Other than that, please keep the hair and scalp clean, wash your locks! And, meticulously care for them by avoiding lint as much as possible. Also, in the beginning I used goo-gobs of a petroleum based 'lock' gel. I would never do that in retrospect. I lost three months of locking due to slippage and unraveling problems, coupled with product flaking. I would have locked with only water, if I knew better.

CREATING BEAUTIFUL LOCKS ON A DIME!

13

Creating Beautiful Locks on a dime

with

Backcombed-Interlocks!

The 3-Step Lock & Roll Method[117]

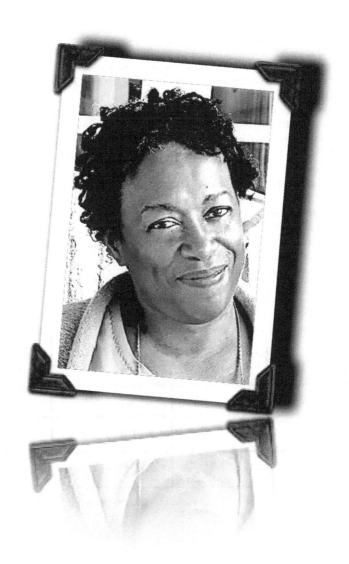

---

[117]Interlocked/crochet/sewed/latched are used interchangeably.

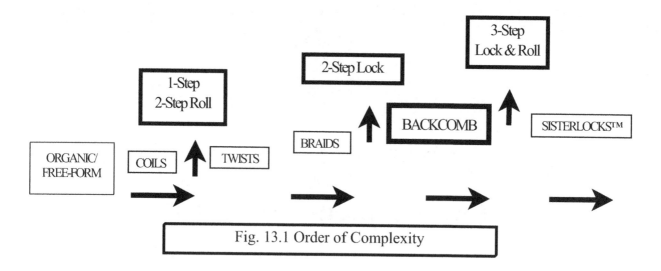

Fig. 13.1 Order of Complexity

Type 1, Type 2 and some Type 3 hair textures are challenging to lock because the texture is predominately made of protein rich keratin in the outer core, which exhibits cuticle behaviors, laying straight, resistant to curls, thus resistant to locking. When considering which foundation to install the loose-haired texture of Type 1 or Type 2, even Type 3, the hair texture has to be the primary concern or the hair will not lock. The straight-haired locker absolutely, must lock the hair intentionally, as the nature of the hair is to unravel and lay straight! To accelerate the locking process, the 3-step lock & roll method is one of the most complicated, necessary installations required to install and secure straight hair into a locked matrix. The initial step backcombing, also known as teasing the hair, occurs when hair is teased incrementally down the length of the hair shaft, from the ends towards the scalp manually or with a comb. Backcombing works because it forces straight hair to knot up and become porous, a trait of highly textured hair, not straight hair; thus, able to mat easily as the cuticles are lifted. For a 2-step lock or 3-step lock & roll method, backcombing will knot the hair near the roots for the initiation of the interlock, because setting the hair into a locked pattern minimizes movement[118]. The interlock is installed from the knot towards the scalp within an eighth of an inch of the scalp, then secured via palm-rolling. Straight haired lockers can successfully maintain their new growth by interlocking the roots in place as the new growth grows in via this method[119]. The ends of the hair are left loose and free, or can be cut away. Some installations only involve backcombing, then palm-rolling. Other techniques may just backcomb the hair and free-form!

Backcomb Methods			
1-Step	2-Step Lock	2-Step Roll	3-Step Lock & Roll
backcombed locks	backcomb	backcomb	backcomb
	interlock	palm roll	interlock
			palm roll

Fig. 13.2 Various backcomb methods

---

[118]The Root of the Matter Chapter

[119]The Root of the Matter Chapter

If the backcomb technique involves palm-rolling, binders like honey, Aloe Vera gel, castor or coconut oil, are used to secure the cylindrical lock formation[120] because they are hydrophilic (dissolves easily in water). The proper balance must be implemented to prevent an ashy appearance from build up that can occur if too much of the binding agent is applied to the lock. Usually, an amount that covers the tip of an index finger is enough for a one inch parting section. However, the amount must be balanced with the locker's individual hair texture. The less dense, the less product needed. The more dense, the more product may be needed. When binders, backcombing and laying an interlocked foundation are used in synergy, the hair mats and the matrix can form as the matted hairs form the net, which is required to begin the integration of the lock foundation at the basic level of infancy. The method used on the model is the 3-step lock & roll method, which incorporates backcombing and interlocking, then palm-roll to secure a locked foundation.

1-Step Method

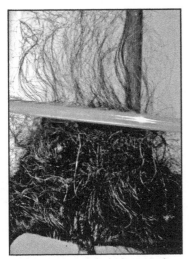

Step 4: Comb hair from ends towards scalp to backcomb.

1. Cleanse locks free of residue, to help the locking process advance.
2. On damp hair, section the hair into the desired pattern, depending upon the desired parting size.
3. Choose a parting design so the dreads will lay on top of one another[121] and secure the other hair away from the section with clips.
4. Backcomb: Slightly twist the hair, then with a small-toothed comb, comb the hair backwards towards the scalp, starting 1 inch from the scalp, then 2 inches from the scalp, then 3...and so on. Comb with one hand. With the other hand, hold the hair tight. After backcombing, inspect the dread and check the hair, repeating until the hair tangles and knots.

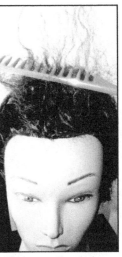

Close up of step four: Comb hair from ends towards scalp to backcomb.

---

[120]The Root of the Matter Chapter

[121]The Parts Chapter

2-Step Lock Method

1. Cleanse locks free of any residue, it will help the locking process advance.
2. On damp hair, section the hair into the desired pattern, depending upon the desired parting size.
3. Choose a parting design so the dreads will lay on top of one another[122] and secure the other hair away from the section with clips.
4. Backcomb: Slightly twist the hair, then comb the hair backwards towards the scalp, starting 1 inch from the scalp, then 2 inches from the scalp, then 3…and so on. Comb with one hand. With the other hand, hold the hair tight. After backcombing, inspect the dread and check the hair.
5. Poke a finger at the base of the backcomb section, then begin the interlock where the knot forms; and, interlock from the knot to the scalp with the tool of choice.

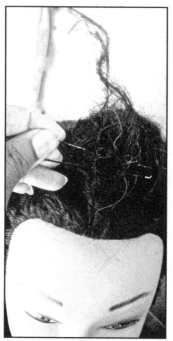

Step 5: Begin the latch from
the knot to the scalp.

---

[122]The Parts Chapter

CREATING BEAUTIFUL LOCKS ON A DIME!

2-Step Roll Method

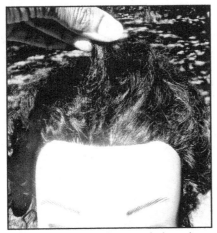

Step 4a: For hard to mat hair, twist hair, then backcomb.

1. Cleanse locks free of any residue, to accelerate the locking process.
2. On damp hair, section the hair into the desired pattern, depending upon the desired parting size.
3. Choose a parting design so the dreads will lay on top of one another[123] and secure the other hair away from the section with clips.
4. On damp hair, backcomb: Slightly twist the hair, then comb the hair backwards towards the scalp, starting 1 inch from the scalp, then 2 inches from the scalp, then 3…and so on. Comb with one hand. With the other hand, hold the hair tight. After backcombing, inspect the dread and check the hair, repeating until the hair tangles and knots.
5. Roll the hair between the fingers or palm of hand, apply the nourishing binding agent to the palms of the hand and palm-roll into the lock[124]. Only apply enough to hold the hairs together[125].

3-Step Lock & Roll Method

1. Cleanse locks free of any residue, to accelerate the locking process(working with dry or wet hair is a preference, find what works best for the locker's hair).
2. On damp hair, section the hair into the desired pattern, depending upon the desired parting size.
3. Choose a parting design so the dreads will lay on top of one another[126] and secure the other hair away from the section with clips.
4. On damp hair, backcomb: Slightly twist the hair, then comb the hair backwards towards the scalp, starting 1 inch from the scalp, then two inches from the scalp, then three…and so on. Comb with one hand. With the other hand, hold the hair tight. After backcombing, inspect the dread and check the hair, repeating until the hair tangles and knots.
5. Poke a finger through the backcomb section, then install the interlock where the knot forms. Interlock the roots in a 4-point rotation[127] from the knot to the scalp.
6. Roll the hair between the fingers or palm of hand, apply the nourishing binding agent to the palms of the hand and palm-roll into the lock[128]. Only apply enough product to hold the hairs together.

---

[123]The Parts Chapter

[124]The Holistic Hair Care Chapter

[125]See *Coils to Locks* section for detailed information

[126]The Parts Chapter

[127]The Root of the Matter Chapter

[128]The Holistic Hair Care Chapter

All of these techniques are done to secure the lock; however, even after installation is complete, the locks may unravel until they are settled. Unraveling is natural and occurs when the hair comes out of its lock formation. This is a natural part of the process, with any texture, during the first few weeks of locking. Backcombed-interlocked locks are complex and can be prone to unraveling, slipping, bunching, frizzing, shrinking and movement among straight hair textures. However, it's the most effective method to lock a dread from a straighter hair texture. As a result, backcombed-interlocked-rolled locks will go through the traditional series of noticeable changes that include bunching, knotting, tangling and condensing. Settling occurs when the hair is left alone, not manipulated and allowed to frizz, knot, tangle and condense without external handling. Settling is an important part of the process during the infancy of the lock foundation, because settling is required for the hair to begin to tangle, mesh, intertwine and knot up, forming the core of the future lock[129]. After palm-rolling this hair type, it's best to dry with a blow drier on a cool setting, or allow to dry in the heat of the sun to avoid mildew build up.

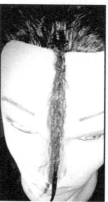

Step 6: The finished look. Interlocked at the roots and palm-rolled down the length of the lock.

---

[129]The Lock Evolution Chapter

Journey
to
Locks
Brenda's Way!

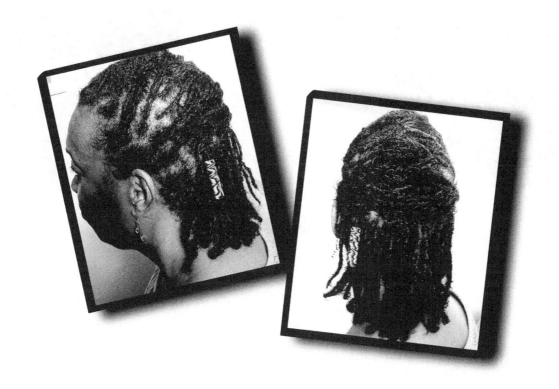

When Brenda began locking she was not particular about the type of locks she preferred. She was flexible and open and loved the simplicity of locks. Because she has a fine Type 2 to Type 3 texture, her lock installation involved the 3-step Lock & Roll technique to secure her fine, straight hair while integrating the curly hair. Brenda has enjoyed her almost two year old locks and has enjoyed the hair regeneration. Brenda is a seasoned locker, locking in her 60's. Due to improper relaxer use, she experienced thinning and partial alopecia in the crown area of her head. As a semi-free former, who only has her roots tool tightened three to four times year, she is a testament to the power of locking the hair and letting the follicles regenerate. Over 60% of her hair has grown back and her once micro-locks have blossomed and filled into beautiful thick, juicy, healthy locks that are brushing her shoulders. The low maintenance allows her flexibility with only quarterly visits to the stylists. She prefers to have her hair tightened, which works well with her schedule. Brenda keeps cost to a minimum by washing with a diluted version of Dr. Bronner's shampoo and Aloe Vera juice spritzes infused with her favorite essential oil. If she uses an oil, she keeps it light with jojoba oil for her less dense hair texture. Now, that's truly locks on a dime!

Infant Locks

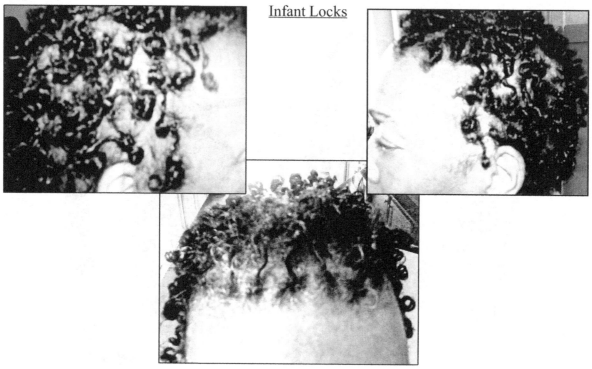

Day 0: Installation locks!

The baby stage was difficult for Brenda because of her loosely textured hair. She experienced a lot of unraveling for the first six months of the journey. She also experienced a lot of part shifting, as her hair follicles generated new hair growth for the first time in years. This shifting meant that her parts changed dramatically as new hair sprouted from once dying follicles. The locks also blossomed and swelled, which required frequent combining within the first eight weeks of her journey. Brenda quickly learned that it was best for her to help her locks mat by spritzing daily with a solution of sea salt or lime juice[130]. After a few minor reinstallation set-backs with unraveling and shrinkage, Brenda was on the way to her new-found journey and a lot of frizz!

---

[130]The Holistic Hair Care Chapter

Teenage Locks

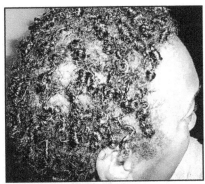

Month 4

Once Brenda's locks settled, she began to enjoy the ease of the whole locking process. She especially loved to extend her tightening sessions even longer now. Unofficially, she became a semi-freeformer. She loved the low maintenance routine; however, it came at a cost as she learned that her scalp became extremely tender, from the lack of daily manipulation. On the contrary, her hair follicles loved it and rewarded her with even more new growth! The tenderness in her scalp caused Brenda to shy away

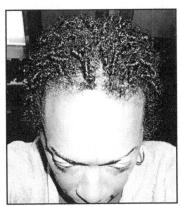

Month 4

from her tightenings even more. Once tightened, she experienced a lot of matting that had to be gently separated at the roots and re-tightened. She loved her routine so much, she continued free-forming. However, she became more fastidious about popping, separating her locks after washing.

Mature Locks

As she approaches year two, Brenda is just entering early maturity. Her hair has expanded greatly; however, her locks have not yet begun to tighten. New growth continues to sprout and her locks are blossoming, growing like weeds, brushing her shoulders. She no longer spritzes with the sea-salt/lime juice; however, she does continue to pop her locks after washing to prevent matting. Brenda loves her mature locks and no longer palm-rolls her now cylindrical locks. The most effort she puts into her hair is tightening the roots, which only takes 50 minutes now by a locktician, once a quarter.

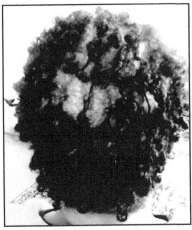

Month 4

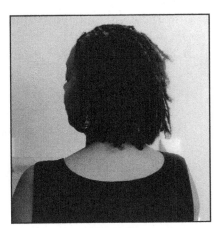

Year 1.5

INTERVIEW

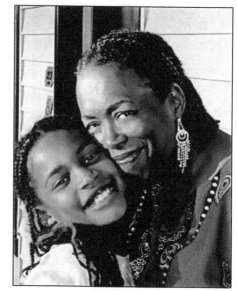

Year 1.5

Name: Brenda Robinson (Mom)
Type of locks: Backcombed-Interlocked-Palm-Rolled
Maintenance: professional latch
2-year-old locks

1. Who was the first person you can recall with locks?

A co-worker over 25 years ago.

2. Did this person influence you to lock?

No

3. What did you think of locks before you locked?

I did not think anything about them.

4. What do you think of locks now?

For me, I think they are the best thing since sliced bread.

5. When you first locked, how did you decide which method would work best for you?

The person who installed them decided this, based on my hair texture.

6. <u>Who helped you decide?</u>

My daughter

7. <u>What was your physical lifestyle before and after locks and how did that change after you locked?</u>

Active lifestyle, this has not changed.

8. <u>Did you begin living a healthier lifestyle after you locked?</u>

Not necessarily

9. <u>How has the maintenance routine of your locks impacted your lifestyle?</u>

I don't have to waste time going to have my hair cut.

10. <u>Did you choose your maintenance routine because of your lifestyle?</u>

Yes.

11. <u>How do you feel about skinny locks?</u>

I like them.

12. <u>How do you feel about big, thick locks?</u>

I like them also, the variety is interesting.

13. <u>How did your feelings about lock size impact your decision to get the lock foundation that you have?</u>

It didn't, I just wanted locks, this had no bearing on this decision.

14. <u>How did the size/diameter of your locks change over the years?</u>

I like all locks, they are interesting.

15. <u>Did your locks seem to condense and grow skinnier with time or did your locks stay the same size?</u>

They condensed, and got thicker and smoother with time; however I'm just going into my second year, so they haven't grown skinnier yet.

16. <u>If a hairstylist respected your time, was at a convenient location with a good environment, would you prefer to get your hair done compared to self-maintenance?</u>

I would prefer someone else doing it.

17. <u>How much is too much to pay for lock installation of traditional locks (twists, braids, coils)?</u>

I think it depends on what your market will bear.

18. <u>How would you describe your personality?</u>

I am outgoing.

19. <u>Do you like to do your own hair?</u>

I love my hair.

20. <u>How much is too much to pay for lock tightening?</u>

I think it depends on what the market will bear.

21. <u>Are your locks heavy?</u>

No, my locks are not heavy at all.

22. <u>Are your locks the size that you envisioned them to be?</u>

I did not care, I just wanted locks.

23. <u>Is there anything you would have done differently your first year of locking, looking back?</u>

I should have separated my locks more after washing them and rinsed better.

14

Creating Beautiful Locks on a Dime!
with
Sisterlocks™!

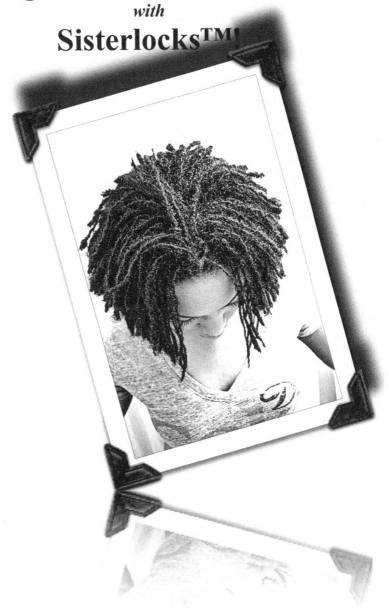

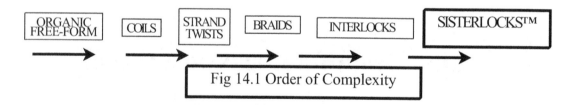

Fig 14.1 Order of Complexity

Sisterlocks™ are small microlocks made with a special trademark tool by Dr JoAnne Cornwell. This technique integrates backward, uniform looping rotations, moving from the ends of the hair towards the scalp. The Sisterlocks™ system is similar to interlocking; however, the patterns, partings and methods are trademarked and implemented with a specialized tightening tool. This technique was developed in the early 1990's and can be installed on chemically straightened hair with at least 1.5 inches of new growth or 100% chemical free hair requiring a professional installation by a certified Sisterlocks™ consultant. The consultant installs 300-800 locks depending upon the size of the head, length of the hairline from front to back, hair texture, hair length, density and parting size preference, all of which directly impact the installation and tightening price. The longer the hair, the higher the price. The thicker the hair, the longer the time, the higher the price as well. There are three sizes: small, medium and large Sisterlocks™, which are also known as Brotherlocks™. The average retightening time for 500 locks can take 2.5 hours if locks are tightened every three to four weeks. With small Sisterlocks™, it is especially important to maintain the fragile root-bed, tightening every three to four weeks, to prevent breakage. Small locks can be more costly than medium to large sized locks because of the time required for installation and maintenance. Medium to large sized locks are stronger and less labor intensive/pricey to install. With time and maturity, the tightening routine can extend beyond six weeks, no longer than eight weeks without compromising the integrity of the locks. Brotherlocks are usually installed on men, but can be installed on women as well. The transformation of Sisterlocks™ will depend upon a person's texture, density and porosity, the key biological traits[131]. As a result, bunching and other irregularities may occur with Sisterlocks™, just like with any other type of lock; however, to a much lesser extent than seen with other, traditional locks. This comprehensive guide will prepare the Sisterlocked individual to participate in the journey by becoming empowered with tips to not only ask the right questions, but to learn how to get Sisterlocks™ on a dime! It is possible!

---

[131]The State of the Hair Chapter

Straight From Chemical Relaxer

to

Sisterlocks™!
Shauna's Story!

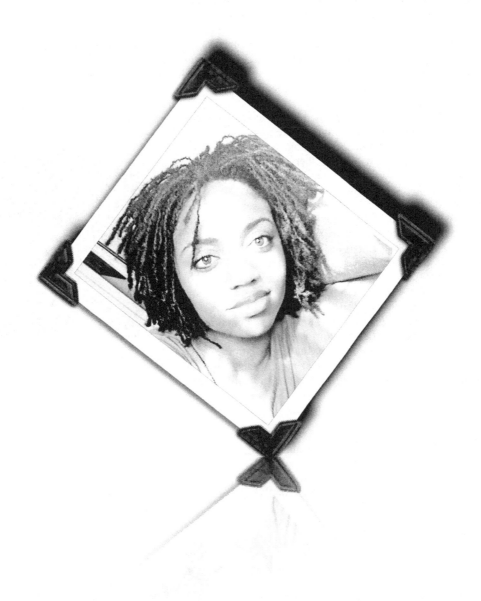

Shauna went straight from chemically relaxed hair to Sisterlocks™ after transitioning for seven months. Shauna learned about the technique and decided to complete her transition to natural hair directly to locks, with her relaxed ends intact. Laborious detangling sessions and the challenges of two textures were not for Shauna with her busy lifestyle as a working mom, and student. The Sisterlocks™ system is high in complexity, setting the bar high for locks as the cadillac of groomed, manicured locks. Because Sisterlocks™ is a technique, with a trademarked tool, they are the most expensive, time consuming and costly of locks to install and to maintain. The beauty of Sisterlocks™ is their ability to look like fine strands of hair. Dr JoAnne Cornwell says that the Sisterlocks™ system is a business that promotes the Sisterlock™ brand offering the flexibility of wash and go hair with styling options[132]. With this in mind, Sisterlocks is a viable option for those desiring this type of installation and maintenance. The beauty of all locks are their versatility and ease of care. Sisterlocks™ offers a brand with an instant community that is networked internationally.

Shauna was concerned about keeping up with the upfront payments and tightenings. She was able to get her Sisterlocks™ on a dime. Instead of choosing a certified consultant, she went to **www.sisterlocks.com** and found a consultant-in-training in her area. To obtain certification, all trainees need to install three different client installations. Because trainees are not certified yet, they may be able to strike a deal, thus, reducing the cost. Weigh the benefits of an experienced, mature certified stylist versus a trainee, carefully. Always ask to see credentials! The Sisterlock™ brand educates consultants that Sisterlocks™ are only certified Sisterlocks™ when the tool is used with the Sisterlocks™ tightening technique. There are many Sisterlockers who have chosen to forge off the beaten path and handle tightenings without the pricey course certification offered to consultants and clients. It's best to weigh the risks with the benefits when deciding how to maintain Sisterlocks™ on a dime, the cost savings may be a benefit; and, it's definitely an option for the confident!

Shauna still opts to have her roots tightened by her consultant. She enjoys the pampering and time it gives her to catch up on her studying, while relaxing. Tightening sessions can range from $25.00-$35.00/hour averaging $60.00/2.5 hour tightening session. Shop around because there are consultants out there that are fair and reasonable, and there are others that will take advantage of the shortage of certified Sisterlock™ consultants and charge much more. The cost of Sisterlocks™ is based upon the chemical-free hair length. Transitioning from a relaxer to Sisterlocks™ or installing them on short hair is another way to keep costs low. Shauna was only charged on her three to four inches of chemical-free hair; therefore, her cost was minimal, making her installation under $500.00. However, clients with twelve inches of chemical-free hair may pay closer to $1000.00 for installation. Shauna also keeps her product cost to a minimum, by sticking with her favorite products: Suave Clarifying Shampoo and Pomegranate Soy Conditioner, Yes to Cucumbers Conditioner and daily Aloe Vera juice spritzes touched with a dash of jojoba and Jane Carter's Leave in Conditioner and rose water. Shauna's locks are a perfect example of how Type 4 hair can mature beautifully from chemically relaxed hair to natural hair with minimal fuss.

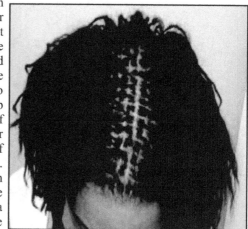

Week 1 Sisterlocks

Infant Locks

For a chemically-relaxed transitioner, like Shauna, locking three to four inches of Type 4 soft, fuzzy hair into small Sisterlocks™ took nineteen hours to install. Shauna's partings were distinct and the grid uniform, which is a unique feature of Sisterlocks™. As long as the locks are tightened in a timely fashion and the root-bed copiously maintained, the partings will remain throughout the lifetime of the Sisterlocks™. Shauna's partings and grid were

[132]Cornwell, JoAnne. *That hair thing: and the Sisterlocks approach*. San Diego, Calif.: Sisterlocks Pub., 1997. Print.

determined by the density of her follicles, texture of her hair, and the density of her hair, as well as her size preference, which was small Sisterlocks™. From there, the size of the grid pattern was set and the parts continued to be fastidiously maintained by tightening every three to six weeks, which depends on her growth cycle.

Shauna was concerned at first because her locks were thin and stiff, at installation, with a lot of scalp showing. That passed as the locks matured, filling in along the scalp. The biological traits[133] will vary for individual lockers. Her follicles are sparse, not dense, thus there was a lot of scalp showing initially. Shauna's consultant assured her that this would pass as once dead follicles would begin regenerating new growth now that the chemical relaxing process was over. She also meticulously continued to care for her two different textures as she carefully transitioned out of her chemical relaxer with Sisterlocks™.

During the first year, the consultant recommended the Sisterlocks™ products for maintenance; because, they are formulated to work with the locks, avoiding heavy, oil-based ingredients with slip in them. Shauna chose to maintain her locks with Suave products and avoided excessive slippage and bunching. There are Sisterlockers that veer off the path and still have a successful journey; however, locking and care can be overwhelming and the designated products and instructions help the consultant care for the Sisterlocks™, while keeping the plan simple for the client. Shauna's consultant was flexible and allowed her to continue using her favorite products. The early days were exciting; yet, nerve wracking, as Shauna balanced feelings of uncertainty with the scalpy look of her roots and her straight chemically-relaxed ends.

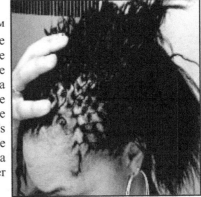

First week

Teenage Locks

As Shauna's locks matured, they expanded, and thickened as her hair began to fill in along the scalp and shed inside of the lock. The baby stage quickly passed away and her hair began to settle. Settling can take from three weeks to six months or longer! During this stage, Shauna avoided bunching and unraveling by avoiding over manipulation of her locks by letting them free-style, and following her consultant's instructions, banding when washing and avoiding detangling conditioners and products with slip. As teenagers, she cared for them by spritzing, moisturizing and feeding the roots, while moisturizing the ends of her hair, because her locks began to mat. She practiced banding and washing her locks the correct way and continued to carefully handle her hair, with the fragile line of demarcation, as she avoided heat and wet-set her straight ends with satin rollers at night or braid-outs.

Month 5
No more relaxed ends!

At seven months, her locks were maturing, and expanding, while the relaxed ends were not looking as attractive, to Shauna. She was finally ready to separate from the chemically treated ends and cut them away from her locks. Unlike traditional locks, Shauna's Sisterlocks™ didn't bud. They began to mesh and condense throughout the core of the lock and thicken.

---

[133]The State of the Hair Chapter

Mature Locks

As Shauna moves toward maturity with her now two-year-old locks, it's time to enjoy and watch her Sisterlocks™ mature and grow! Mature Sisterlocks™ will look very differently than installed Sisterlocks™. Mature Sisterlocks™ are two to three times larger, regardless of the installed size. They will continue to become uniform, settled, tight and compact throughout. Shauna can expect to see more growth as she grows with her locks.

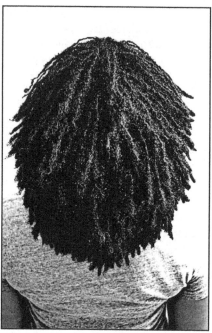

Newly mature locks
year 2.0

INTERVIEW

Name: Shauna Hollinger (~GAN~)
Type of locks: Sisterlocks™
Maintenance: Sisterlocks™ tool tightening by a
consultant every 5-6 weeks
2-year-old locks

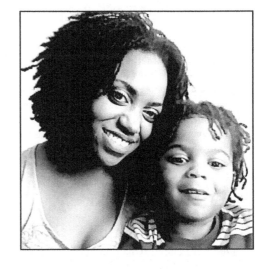

1. Who was the first person you can recall with locks?

My aunt has locks which she started with extensions. That was the first person in real life that I knew. Other than that, I stumbled upon a girl that goes by Kalia Dewdrop on www.blogspot.com and I was hooked on her hair. She had Sisterlocks™ at the time (now traditional) and I emailed her about them. My interest took off from there.

2. Did this person influence you to lock?

Not so much my aunt, but some women on www.nappturality.com did. The blogs inspired me the most. I had never seen so many different kinds of locks and didn't know there were so many ways to to do them.

3. What did you think of locks before you locked?

To be honest, I had a very stereotypical way of thinking about them. I felt like you had to be "afrocentric" or a Rasta to wear locks. I'm so embarrassed by that. I really wasn't exposed to many people who had them. I grew up in a white area and saw very few natural people at all. By the time I moved to a predominately black area, I started seeing a few more naturals. Surprisingly, I see more naturals with locks at my job and I work for the government. To me it's odd because I see more natural women in a business setting rather than just out and about.

4. What do you think of locks now?

I LOVE all kinds of locks now! I've seen every kind and have fell in love with each type. Free-form, braidlocks, Sisterlocks™, etc. I love them all. I think they each have their own unique beauty. Now that I have a better understanding of natural hair altogether, the stereotypes I had in my mind are long gone and I see all kinds of people wearing them.

5. When you first locked, how did you decide which method would work best for you?

I was still transitioning and really started thinking about what was I going for or trying to achieve. Length? Healthy hair? Something easy to manage? When I got to my 7th month of transitioning, I was so sick of dealing with the two textures but I wasn't ready to chop yet. I wanted to transition for at least 12-15 months. When I found out that you could start locks with permed ends by doing Sisterlocks,™ that was all I needed to know. It gave me the best of both worlds at the time. It allowed me to continue to transition, not worry about struggling with both textures, I didn't have to stress out about figuring out how to style my hair (I didn't know how to do that anyway), and someone else essentially was going to be doing my hair which left little for me to have to do except wash and separate. At the time, I thought that was the ONLY way to start locks with relaxed ends though. Had I known I could have done the same with braidlocks, I probably would have gone that route instead.

6. Who helped you decide?

My husband helped me decide. Actually, he told me about Sisterlocks™ long before I even went natural. He suggested I chop my hair and go natural when he saw all the issues I was having with my hair. I thought he was crazy because in my mind, I would be ugly if I did that. I didn't think he knew what he was talking about when he mentioned Sisterlocks™, so I ignored him because I had been told that it was impossible to start locks without being 100% natural. When I brought Sisterlocks™ back up, he was all for it.

7. What was your physical lifestyle before and after locks and how did that change after you locked?

My physical lifestyle was not very active. I was scared to mess up my hair or sweat out my perm before going natural. Now that my hair is already "done" everyday, I don't have to worry about any of that. I can wash my hair whenever I want and I go on about my day. I spend no time at all doing my hair now. I may finger comb or spray my hair with water and that's it. I've got 30 minutes of my morning back!

8. Did you begin living a healthier lifestyle after you locked?

Yes. I'm not sure that being locked had much to do with it as much as me starting to have health issues due to my eating habits. That is what really made me start being healthier. Working out has become more enjoyable and I don't worry about my hair anymore when I do. I can finally focus on the workout and not messing up my hair.

9. How has the maintenance routine of your locks impacted your lifestyle?

It's impacted my lifestyle by allowing me to have more time to do other things in the mornings before I go to work, less saturdays are spent in the salon, less time is spent in the salon, and less money is spent on hair.

10. Did you choose your maintenance routine because of your lifestyle?

Yes. I have a toddler, I take online classes part time for school, and I work full time. I wouldn't have time to retighten my own hair. I do know how in case I ever have to though. I enjoy going to the salons just to get time to myself and get away from the house for a couple hours. Also, getting locks, was something I wanted to do so I could have less maintenance because of my lifestyle. I didn't want my hair to consume my life as it did before I went natural.

11. How do you feel about skinny locks?

I like skinny locks! I always liked thinner locks for myself even though I think the thicker ones look amazing on people. I loved the pictures I would see of really long Sisterlocks™. As time went on, I started to like medium or slightly thicker locks even more. I will probably combine them later on down the road after I have them for awhile.

12. How do you feel about big, thick locks?

I love those too. I didn't feel like they would fit me and my personality, but there are some ladies on www.nappturality.com that have big thick locks and look amazing. Bajanempress being one of them. The model Nerissa Irving looks amazing with her thick locks as well.

13. How did your feelings about lock size impact your decision to get the lock foundation that you have?

I never really had a strong feeling about lock size one way or another. I just knew I wanted my hair to be locked. It wasn't so much the size that impacted my decision, but more so the method and how soon I could get them.

14. How did the size/diameter of your locks change over the years?

Looking back on the pictures from when I first got them installed, they have expanded maybe two or three times the size they originally were.

15. Did your locks seem to condense and grow skinnier with time or did they stay the same size?

They have condensed, but they have grown thicker. The ends especially have gotten rather thick.

16. If a hairstylist respected your time, was at a convenient location with a good environment would you prefer to go to get your hair done compared to self-maintenance?

For now, I'd prefer to get them done being that I have a really busy schedule. Its also nice because I view it as being pampered. My consultant is less than ten minutes away from my home, she's fast, she has a really nice salon, and she does a fantastic job. I wouldn't have it any other way right now. If I ever move, I will probably just do them on my own.

17. How much is too much to pay for lock installation of traditional locks(twists, braids, coils)?

I think Sisterlocks™ are expensive upfront, but looking at the time it takes and how precise it is when getting them installed, I can understand. I've heard of some people charging $1,000 for Sisterlocks™. At the same time someone could say me paying $480 was ridiculous too. The reason why I'm ok with it is because it's a one time thing and I never have to pay that much again. In my mind, it was no different than me paying for micro-braids and or a weave over and over, except smarter since it was a one time thing. If I maintained my own locks, I'd save even more money, but not time, and that is really important to me. I was spending about $200 a month before I went natural/got locks. Paying for Sisterlocks™ ended up being more of a money saver to me than anything despite the high cost upfront.

18. How would you describe your personality?

I'm a pretty friendly person and eager to help others, especially when it comes to natural hair.

19. Do you like to do your own hair?

I do like doing my own hair, although I don't know how to do many styles. If I do anything, it will be very basic. I normally wear it up or down. I may even throw a flower in my hair on special occasions but that's about it! I wish I knew how to do more styles, but that's one of the reasons why I love locks because you don't have to do anything to them in order for them to look good.

20. How much is too much to pay for lock tightening?

I think it depends on the person. Some people are willing to pay a lot of money but "a lot of money" is defined differently by different people. I pay $25 an hour which normally comes to about $50-$65 every 5-6 weeks. Anything more than that would be steep to me. At the same time, I may even be willing to pay more since it saves me so much time from not having to do it myself.

21. Are your locks the size that you wanted them to be, looking back?

Yes they are! I'm actually surprised that they are as big as they are right now. I like the size!

22. Is there anything you would have done differently?

My tip would be to research all kinds of methods of starting locks before committing to one. Think about if you want to continue going to a locktician or if you want to do it on your own. Then, consider the time it takes to do them on your own and the price if you want to get it done by a locktician.

I love my Sisterlocks™ and I love that I was able to start them with permed ends, but I could have started them the same way with braids to get a similar look. I probably would have gone that route had I known. I was able to go to someone who knew what she was doing and I knew she was trained. There was no guessing on how my hair was going to look. I would also suggest looking at different blogs and pictures of others with the same type of hair density that you have along with the different lengths so you can compare what yours might look like.

Knotty Note

How to Grow Sisterlocks™ on a Dime!

1. Choose medium/large Sisterlocks™
2. Install on 1.5-3 inches of virgin hair
3. Install on chemically free hair under 5 inches in length
4. Consider a Sisterlocks™ consultant-in-training
5. Strike a deal with a consultant
6. Take the Sisterlocks™ tightening course for self-maintenance
7. Use other products with low slip for maintenance
8. Discuss the average price of the work nationwide, and work a deal

Beautiful Mature Sisterlocks™[134]

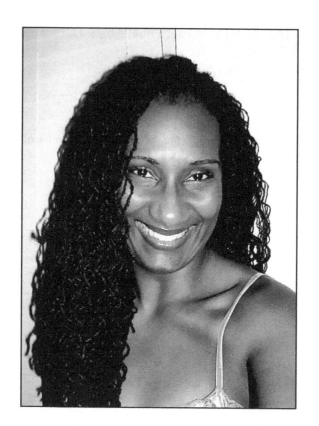

---

[134]Bena's Seasoned, mature Sisterlocks™ older than 5 years. This style is called a braid-out.

Black Girls Do Swim!

I never liked to be splashed on with water or to get my face wet. Quite simply, if my face got wet, my hair got wet. If my hair got wet, then there was drama. And there isn't a swimming cap that I know of that is worth its price. Once emerged in the water, my swimming caps always transformed into a mini swimming pool for my hair. The only benefit it served was to contain my fro. There were two choices: Swimming cap, to contain the napps, or wear it loose and risk looking like an ashy version of Buckweet from The Little Rascals, sigh. Both options were lacking, to me. So for more

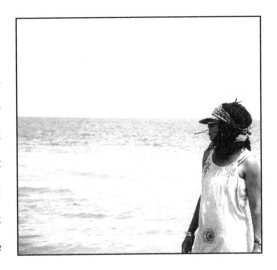

decades than I care to divulge, I have pushed my swimming skills to the side and opted to float with noodles, boogie boards and other floating devices, while trying to stay away from kids that splash. But, this summer I had to test the waters. I was floating along fine in the Gulf, believe it or not. In Mid Florida, oil had not made its way to the beaches and I had to get to the beautiful Gulf waters one more time, just in case. I went into the ocean with my boys and was peacefully feeling the salt waters massage my muscles and take away years of tension, stress and toxicity from my body. Then, out of nowhere a big giant wave had the nerve to slap me upside the back of my head!

All of those old feelings of 'water fear' came back upon me as I screamed "MY HAIR" my boys laughed at me as they teased me and taunted that I have locks now, I'm supposed to be able to get my hair wet now. They had no clue how long it took to set those curls in my locks for our vacation; however, I laughed too, they were right. The old thinking had not left me. "Because my cute curls are all gone!" They laughed, I laughed, and knew I looked silly and I was astonished that I still held onto the same issues I had as a child with chemical-free hair, regarding water. I swam and felt my locks float to the top of the water. It was an amazing feeling. I felt my hair hug my shoulders as I came up from the water. I was doing all the swim moves that I learned decades earlier; and, I felt muscles move that I haven't felt in years and I felt my locks singing!!! The excitement of being locked and natural came upon me like never before. It took me back to the days when I hated to get my hair washed. Washing was a long process with my long type 4b/4c/z hair. There were the long fights with my napps and the comb, the snapping tangles and knots, the pain. Then there was the detangling session afterwards and more of the same fights with the comb, the snapping, the tangles and knots and the pain. Then, there was the china bump session-what we affectionately now call nubian curls or afro knots. We would not be caught DEAD with those things in our head in the 70's! It was a sign that the beautification process was not complete and the hot comb was coming. The hot comb meant more fights with the comb, the knots, the napps, the pain AND the heat; the sizzle of the blue afro sheen hair grease and the predictable burns followed by cocoa butter and vaseline treatments for weeks before the permanent badge of honor set it, the brown mark or scar. By the time the hairdo was done, everyone was cranky, tired and in some kind of pain. Water and hair were not words synonymous with good times up in my house. Torture sessions were more like it.This summer, I swam for the first time, uninhibited. Water became my friend and I look forward to swimming in the ocean, God willing, again. Black girls do Swim! At least this one does!

PART FOUR

LOCK MANAGEMENT

How To Style on a Dime!
Accessorizing and Styling

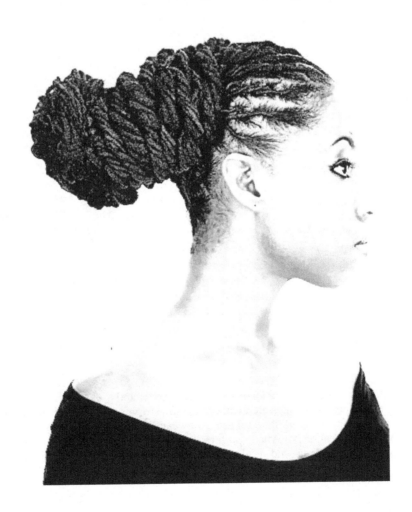

There is a misconception that locks are boring, always look the same, have limitations. This misconception could not be further from the truth. Accessorizing locks is not hard. One of the most beautiful aspects of locks is they are their own accessories. Locks can be tied into bows, swirled into curls and pulled into straight lines that pierce into the air forming aesthetic pieces of art. There are very practical ways to make locks beautiful, dynamic, stylish, practical and trendy. The only limitation is the mind's possibilities. Accessorizing and styling locks are the key. Accessories can be dressed up in the form of doodads, trinkets, ribbons, bows, and yes even hair extensions to create stunning looks that fit the mood of any occasion.

Accessorizing

Accessorizing can be as simple as ABC with original, one-of-a-kind pieces created by entrepreneurs like Mimi, the creator of Tomoka's Twists found online at www.tomokastwists.com. Tomoka's Twists was established for the desire of the growing number of women embracing their natural hair to creatively and functionally adorn their crowns. Tomoka's Twists are flexible, comfortable, and unique. Mimi makes it simple to coordinate outfits with fashionable hair designs because of the unique care she puts into creating each piece. As a Certified Sisterlock™ Consultant, Mimi is in touch with her customer's needs, hailing from North Carolina and shipping her gems around the world.

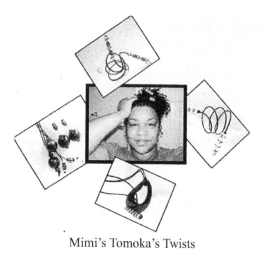

Mimi's Tomoka's Twists

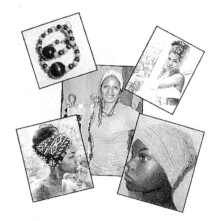

Vanessa's Virtuous Creations

All days are not good hair days, some days it may be necessary to cover and protect the locks. When that day comes, accessorizing with scarves and head coverings are invaluable. Satin scarves can be purchased at beauty supply stores or created from beautiful, colorful fabric. If short on time, they can be purchased directly online from vendors such as Vanessa, owner of Virtuous Creations of Atlanta at http://www.vcreations.biz. She has 'chic and unique' natural hair accessories plus lock jewelry, rings, and headbands, scarves and hats to perk up a challenging lock day for women and men.

So, you still claim you just don't know what to do with your hair? There is no excuse with beautiful lock jewelry available on www.etsy.com and various natural hair sites, they are everywhere[135]! Inspirations by Robin on etsy.com boasts of beautiful hair beads that can be used to adorn braids or locks at http://www.etsy.com/people/LuvingYourLocks. Funky purses, hats, shoes and belts crocheted by Gwen can add to individual flavor and flair. Gwen's designs can be found at http://www.gwenjbags.com.

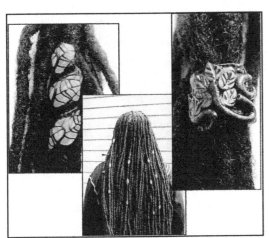

Robin's LovinYourLocks

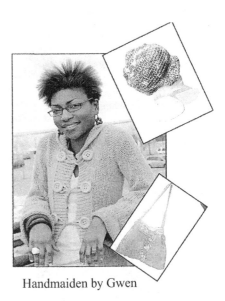

Handmaiden by Gwen

These designs are just a few examples of the options that are available for natural hair and locks. The following accessories can additionally be used to create styles with flare and attitude[136]. Make it work!

[135]Google lock jewelry

[136]Make your own hair ties on youtube.

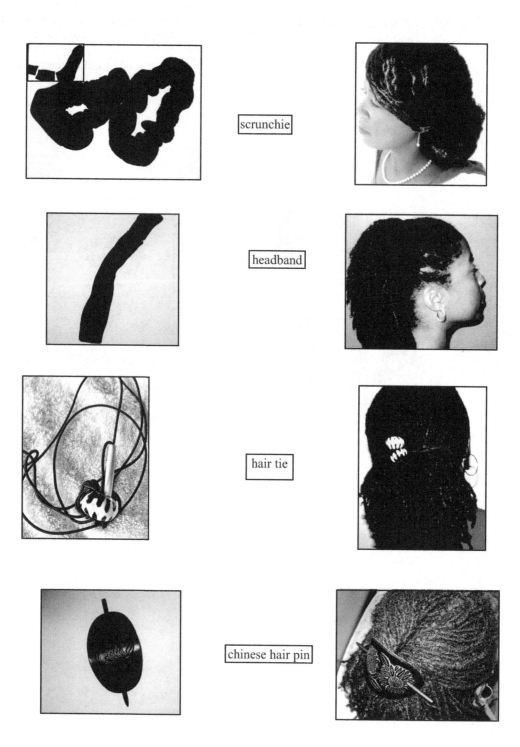

scrunchie

headband

hair tie

chinese hair pin

Still not convinced of the lock possibilities? Cover it up with a hat then, or wrap it up in a scarf[137]!

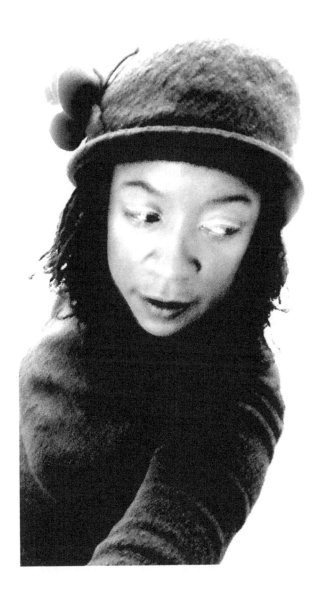

<hr />

[137]Find demos online by doing a google search.

Yes, locks are versatile. Now, it's time to decide how to style the locks, while letting them grow free! Lock styles can be intricate and bold or simple and crisp. We share five core styles that will lead to endless possibilities[138] with Up-Do's buns, curls, swirls, hang-time, braids and plaits.

- Up-Do's
- Buns
- Curly-Do's
- Bantu Knots
- Straight
- Braids/Plaits
- Children's hairstyles

---

[138]YouTube provides step by step, detailed demonstrations on many styles listed.

STYLES

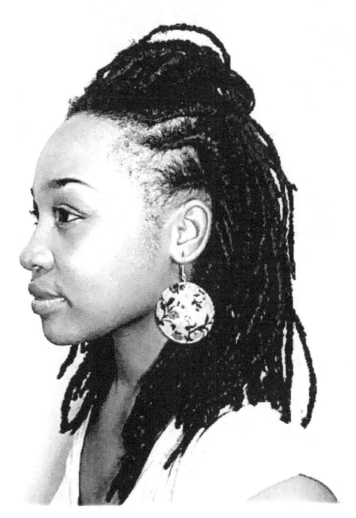

Straight Locks Styled

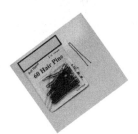 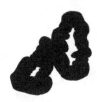

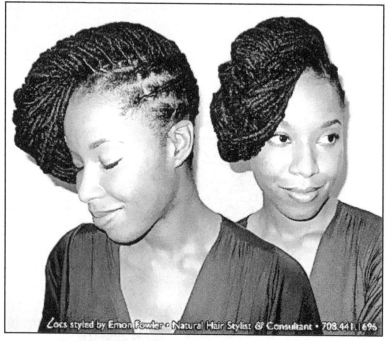

This lovely up-do is done by Emon Fowler who
integrates a fish tail up-do with twists on the side.

The Up-Do

The Up-Do can be done so many ways; and the most beautiful combination up-do's integrate buns, braids, twists, or bantu knot combinations, creating beautiful designs that upsweep the hair away from the face. The main staples for an up-do are hair pins[139], mesh hair nets and fingers to mold the up-do into perfect place. Locks can be integrated with a creative basket weave or a classy roll, secured with hair pins, clips, hair extensions or tied in knots. Let the imagination take you to unchartered waters of many possibilities!

1. Hair net (to blend in and capture loose locks)
2. 2.5 inch hair pins
3. Scrunchie (if needed)

---

[139] A 2.5 inch hair pin is best for locks. Hair pins are not bobby pins!

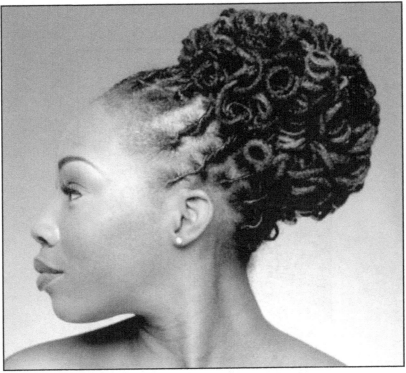

The Bun

The bun can be fun. It can be off to the side, on top of the head, to the back, hang low, loose, curly, braided, twisted, knotted tucked under or placed into a chignon. The main staples for the bun are scrunchies, hair pins, a hair net and satin scarf to smooth down the edges if necessary. If the locks are too short for a bun, hair ties can be used to give the illusion of a full bun, secured with a hair net for fullness. Don't forget to accessorize it with a feathered head-band, scarf, flower, hair beads, sticks, extension hair or ribbons to dress it up!

1. Scrunchie (or hair tie)
2. Hair net
3. Hair pins
4. Extension hair

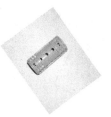 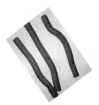 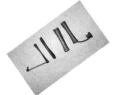

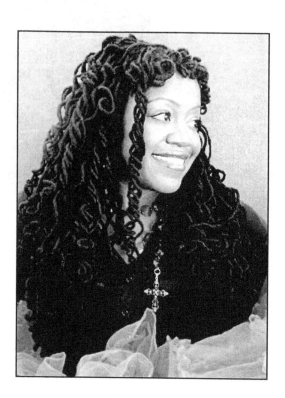

The Curly-Do

When it's time to add a curl, the options are endless. Go old school curling locks with strips of paper bags, foam rollers, perm rods, straws, foam rollers, hard rollers, hair pins, pillow-cushion rollers, and even pipe cleaners aka chenille sticks! The key to a tight curl is to roll only two to three locks per roller on soaping wet hair. The size of the roller matters as well. The smaller the roller, the tighter and smaller the curl. The larger the roller, the looser and bouncier the curl. The more locks put on the roller, the looser the curl, the fewer the locks on a roller, the smaller and tighter the curl. Just remember, tight, small curls can last for days. Loose, bouncy curls may last only for 3-4 days at the most. Put in all the curls you like. The absolute *best* setting lotion for locks is water ' bar-non'; however, try out Aloe Vera gel for a strong hold, as well. Simply coat the lock with this water-based gel and roll.

How to Use Lock Curlers

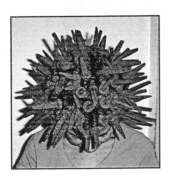

1. Start wrapping the end of the lock near the end with the loop.

2. After the lock is secure with one or two wraps, start rolling/winding the lock up toward the pointed end. Continue until the lock is curled to the scalp.

3. Insert the pointed end of the curler into the loop and pull tight to lock the curler in place.

4. Make sure the hair is COMPLETELY dry before unwinding the hair from the curler[140].

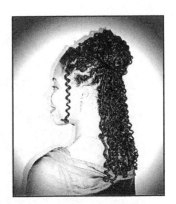

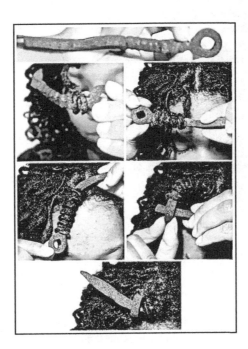

---

[140]Can also be done on similar rollers of another name for the spiral, crinkly look.

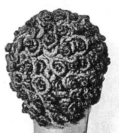

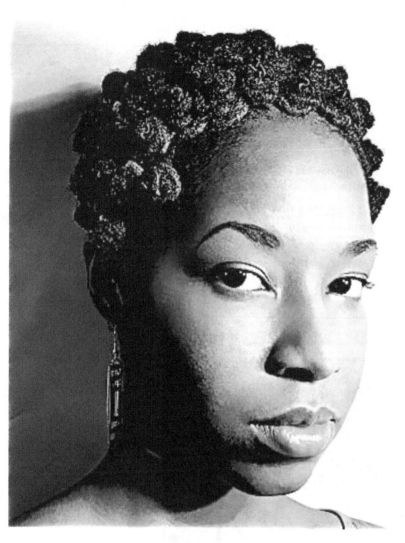

Bantu Knots

Bantu Knots, also known as china bumps, are made by twisting the hair in a single coil or a double-stranded coil into a circular formation, then securing along the scalp by tucking the ends of lock under or with a hair pin. There is no right or wrong way to do them. Just intertwine the hair into a small 'cinnamon bun' at the scalp and secure. Some lockers will choose to wear their coils as bantu knots for the first year, never letting them loose until after year one. The hair is washed, dried and worn like this continuously for the first year as a method to lock the hair. This method works best on highly textured hair. For a simple style, bantu knots can be worn as-is or used to set the hair, then released into a loose wavy hair style. Pin them up and even let them hang, after setting the hair, for a wavy look.

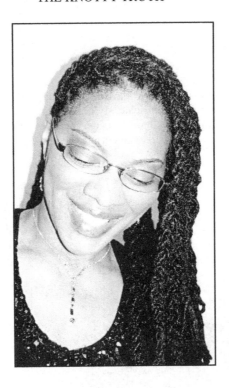

Braids and Twists

To set a wavy look, without the addition of curlers, locks can be set into intricate patterns of waves with braids or twists. The longer the braid/twist set is left in, the longer the curl pattern will remain. When the hair is wet or with time and gravity, the waves will eventually drop. A tight pattern set for at least a week on sopping, wet hair can last up to two weeks. Simply place the locks into plaits or strand twists, leave them in for a day up to a week, then release for a wavy look. Try different patterns of plaited braids or twists and boxed braids or boxed twists until the desired look is achieved, on damp or wet hair. The wetter the hair, the longer the set, the tighter the crinkle.

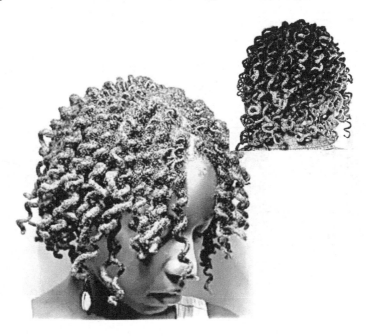

Styles for The Little Ones

Little girls look beautiful with locks. The beauty of locks is the hair style flexibility without tangles! Another great reason to lock a little one's head is because little girls grow into young ladies, then women, who want hair styles similar to their counterparts with up-do's and intricate styling designs. Instead of getting expensive extensions installed throughout the year or damaging healthy hair, consider locking during child hood for long hair with styling options, that can range from pony tails to bangs and even curly styles. The possibilities are endless.

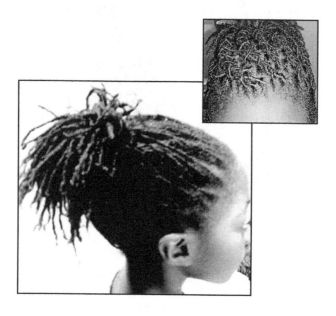

Little boys also grow locks and have just as many styling options. Whether swimming, climbing, playing or styling, locks are an alternative that's easy on the budget, and saves time for everyone in the family.

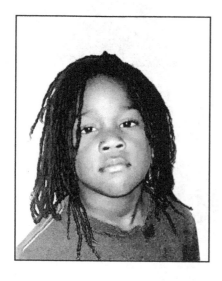

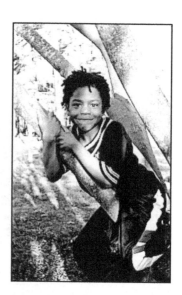

Protect Locks!

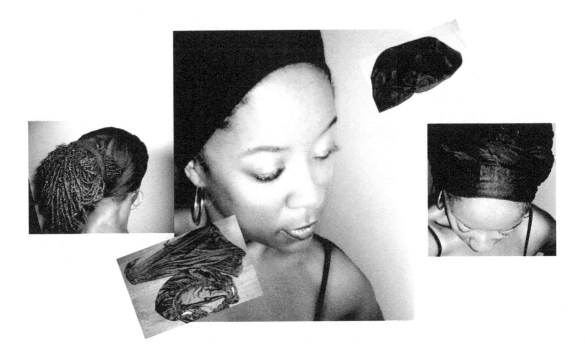

After the style is set it's just as important to protect the style. At night, protect locks with a satin scarf free of elastic around the headband, to prevent premature balding along the hair line. Before putting on a hat, line and protect locks with a satin turban scarf as shown in The Lock Challenge Chapter. In the shower, cover up locks with shower caps made especially to compensate for large locks. Regular shower caps will work fine for small to medium length locks. For extra protection, while sleeping, cover pillows with a satin pillowcase to protect the skin and hair from dehydration!

CREATING BEAUTIFUL LOCKS ON A DIME!

The Great Lock
Take Down!

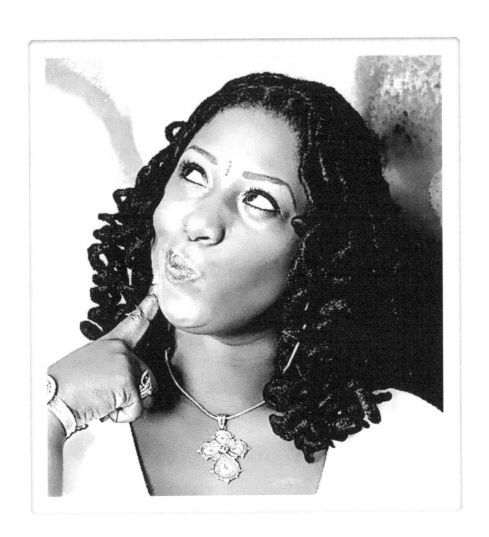

There may come a time for a lock journey to end. If that time should come, there are different ways to take locks down. It takes commitment and patience to grow locks; however, it only takes a moment to get rid of them. It's important to be aware of the impact if the decision has been made to eliminate the locks. This process is usually difficult on loved ones, friends, coworkers requiring a period of adjustment and acceptance for all. Locks really do impact the community.

The reasons for cutting locks may vary. Some share that they desire to release negative energy from a painful life experience: the death of a loved one, end of a marriage, abuse or depression. Others seek a change in lifestyle and simply wish to start anew. There are still societal stigmas attached to locks, causing some to co-opt to a *clean-cut corporate look* for gainful employment, this pressure is often felt by men. Some lockers simply are dissatisfied with the appearance of their locks and want to start over. Finally, some lockers find themselves in the midst of alopecia, hair-thinning-from trauma to the body, from medical procedures such as child birth, surgery, or simple stress. Physical trauma is harmful because stress-induced hormones are released within the body, while chemicals used for surgery can manifests through hair-loss and dermatological conditions as they work their way out of the body for up to a year post event. This trauma, whether induced or natural, can manifest as root-thinning or thinning along the shaft of the lock, or both.

Knotty Note

Reasons to Release the Locks and Start Again

1. Release negative energy from bad experiences

2. Change lifestyle

3. Dissatisfaction with appearance

4. Employment

5. Alopecia/hair thinning from medical procedures like postpartum, surgery

Once the decision has been made, there is more than one way to take down locks. The easy way is to cut the locks off immediately. The hard way, involves picking the locks out. The decision will depend on lifestyle and personal preference, as all methods have their advantages and disadvantages. Regardless of the method chosen, this process is usually frightening, exciting and daunting all at the same time, as this step marks the beginning of another journey and learning process to loose, natural hair that is a totally different journey[141].

---

[141] Read the first book of The Knotty Truth series by George, M. Michele. *The Knotty Truth: Managing Tightly Coiled Hair at Home*. 2nd ed. Columbus, Ohio: Manifest Publishing Enterprises, 2007. Print.

DE-LOCKING METHODS

METHOD	ADVANTAGE	DISADVANTAGE
Grow-Out	More options with remaining hair length	Patience as hair grows out, root tension
Cut-Out	Quick	No hair
Pick-Out	Hair retention	Tedious, time consuming process, damaged hair

Fig. 16.1

GROW OUT

Growing locks out involves patience. For those who wish to have length, growing the hair out two to four inches will allow the former locker to exercise style options once the locks are gone. While growing out the loose new-growth, it is perfectly fine to brush the new-growth with a soft boar head brush, during the in-between stage, being careful to not tear at any creepers or married locks. In fact, it's best to continue popping and separating the roots and fastidiously care for the roots with frequent nourishment and massages, to keep the hair healthy, preventing matting at the roots. After a while, there is stress between the new-growth and the lock which may manifest as thinning roots, requiring the locks to finally be cut away. Once the locks are cut away, this hair will be exposed to climate changes and styling manipulation; therefore, it's best to prepare a healthy head of hair to start with building a strong foundation into the new transition phase, while strengthening the tender scalp that is no longer used to manipulation. There will be a period of soreness. Nourishing massages help to stimulate blood flow and strengthen the scalp[142] which is critical for healthy hair.

Tools:

•Scrunchie
•Scissors
•Cleanser
•Deep Conditioning Treatment
•Pick/comb
•Towel

---

[142]The Lock Challenge Chapter

Directions:

1. Pull locks away from the scalp one at a time.

2. Cut the locks at the line of demarcation where the loose roots meet the lock.

3. Pick out any remaining matted hair at the top of the new-growth or simply trim it away.

4. Wash the hair with a good moisturizing cleanser and follow up with a deep moisturizing treatment, trim and style the hair.

CUT-OUT

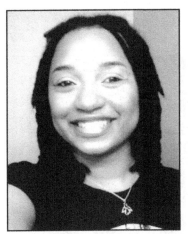

Ya-akura did a combination cut-out grow-out with her 3-year-old locks

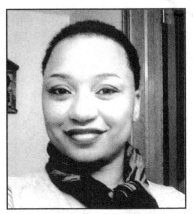

After the Cut-Out

The quickest way to get rid of locks is to cut them at the roots, shaving the head bald. This is often an option for those undergoing chemotherapy, the impatient or the brave.

Tools:

- Scissors
- Shaving Cream
- Clippers
- Wash Cloth
- Towel
- Cleanser
- Jojoba Oil

Directions:

1. Cut the locks off at the roots.
2. Apply shaving cream to the head.
3. Shave any remaining hair on the head off.
4. Clean the scalp, then massage jojoba oil to nourish and feed the follicles and scalp.

PICK OUT

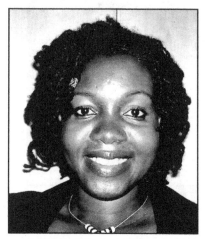

Ofo's braidlocks before take - down

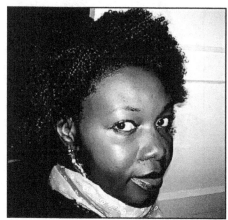

After the lock take-down

One of the most frustrating methods to release locked hair is to pick each lock apart one by one. For some, it is more difficult to unravel interlocked locks than palm-rolled locks, because the hair is matted into locked loops. For others, interlocks take longer. Regardless of the maintenance technique chosen, it is a tedious, long process not to be taken lightly. Hours must be devoted to this process, that can lead to days. Necks, fingers, backs, arms will be exhausted when the process is complete; and, the hair will be in poor shape. The hair will be damaged simply from the take-down process, the picking and prodding to free the hair. The hair will be thinner, may feel extremely dry and in need of a desperate trim. Most of the hair will be shed hair, resulting in a grocery bag full of hair or more at the end of the take-down process, so don't be surprised! Remember, locks are the formation of matted, shed hair, and that shed hair will come out now that the matrix of the lock is released. Taking supplements such as biotin, drinking water and eating healthy vegetables and Omega-3 rich fatty foods can help to rebuild the hair.

Tools:

•A tool to pick the locks apart: sharp pin, safety, needle, fork, paper clip, end of a rat-tail comb, cable stitch needle...
•Scissors
•Cleanser
•Towel
•Take-Out Mixture[143] (warm 10 seconds in microwave):
> 1 tbspn ACV
> 2 oz creamy conditioner
> 4 oz water
> microwave safe cup
> holding dish

---

[143]Remake mixture as needed. If preferred, some commercial product lines sell take down solutions.

Directions:

1. Saturate locks with take-out mixture overnight, cover head with a shower cap, secure with a scarf.

2. In the morning, dunk first lock in the take-out mixture.

3. With the scissors, cut the tip of the lock off or begin to unravel at the tip with tool of preference.

4. Pick the lock out from the end of the lock towards the scalp.

5. Secure each section with a braid or 2-strand twist.

6. Wash the hair with a good moisturizing cleanser and follow up with a deep moisturizing treatment, trim and style the hair.

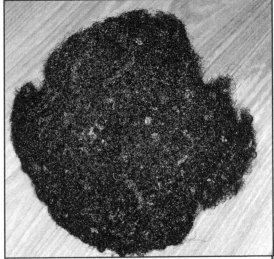

Shed hair from the take-down.

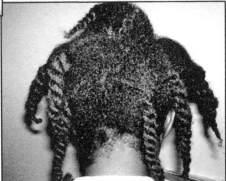

Secure hair for washing after take-down.

CREATING BEAUTIFUL LOCKS ON A DIME!

FINDING THE
RIGHT
STYLIST

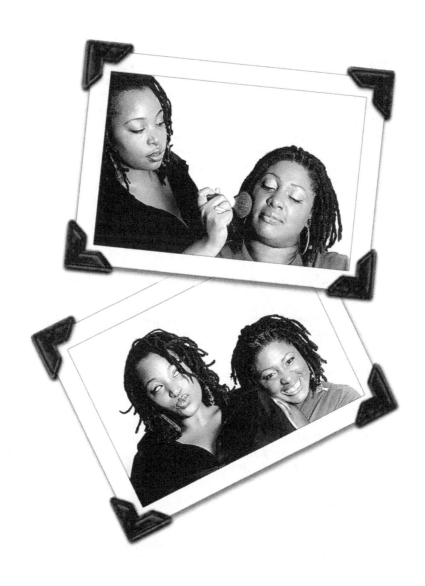

Doing-It-Yourself/Self-Maintenance is not for everyone because some clients may want the care of a professional due to physical limitations, personal preference and/or the need for simple guidance throughout the locking process. When looking for someone to work on locks, look for someone credible in the care of natural hair first, secondly look for someone experienced with the care of locks. A stylist experienced with locks may have different titles; and, the key is to have someone care for locks that has gone the extra mile to learn the art of locking. The following are common names used by those who care for locks:

- Locktician
- Beautician
- Cosmetologist
- Hair Dresser
- Natural Hair Stylist
- Natural Hair Consultant
- Loc Specialist
- Sisterlock™ Consultant

Not everyone with a licensed title can do this job. Because the care of highly textured hair is often learned beyond the walls of traditionally beauty schools, it's important to be diligent and do the research required to find the best person for the job! The first step is to be diligent and take time to do the research with an initial consultation to evaluate the condition of the hair and gather background information from the stylist and *for* the client. Take the time to thoroughly interview the stylist with questions. While gathering information, be aware that today most natural hair stylists are usually not licensed. Unfortunately, the Managing Cosmetology standardized test for licensed hair professionals does not test on chemical-free-Afro-textured hair, beyond ground zero which is straight hair. As a result, many stylists experienced in the care of natural hair do not attend traditional schools of learning and may be self-taught or certified through an alternative program. Consequently, it's vitally important to do the homework and ask the right questions, because this expanding field of hair care is often found off the traditional beaten path. The following questions are important to ask when deciding who is the best stylist to install and care for locks:

Provider Questions

Are you licensed or certified and where did you get your experience with natural hair care?

Remember the key is 'experience' when it comes to natural hair care, because it is not taught in cosmetology school. Listen for best practices and care of the hair, asking to see pictures of clients and styles.

What kind of locks do you have the most experience with?

Remember there are many different methods to start locks with. Some stylists may shun one method over another, because of lack of experience, not because the method is poor. If you are resolved in the method you want, gently share this manual with them and your resources to steer them on the right path. However, it is fine to trust in the stylist's abilities. Stay cognizant of the fact that an opinion does not make a method a poor method, it just is not the preference of that particular stylist; and, unfortunately, they chose words that are a deterrent.

Do you use heat to dry the hair after washing?

Heat damages the bonds within the cortex of the hair. Heat can permanently damage the hair regardless of the 'protectant' used by the stylists. If possible, sit under a hooded dryer and ask to have hair blown dry on a non-

heated setting, or take your satin scarf cap with you to the hairdresser, cover the hair, Then put a hat or bandana on and leave when services are complete, letting the hair dry naturally. This may become difficult in the winter-time because of extreme cold. If this is the case, a cool setting using a blow-drier or hooded-drier is acceptable as long as hair care is complimented with deep oil treatments while under the care of the locktician. Yes, oil can set the locking process back; however, it's more important to give the hair the nourishment it requires to prevent damage that can lead to dry, brittle locks that snap off.

What tools do you use for lock maintenance and installation?

At installation, hair should only be detangled on damp hair, free of oils with a large-toothed rounded comb or a large toothed brush. After brushing, secure hair in sections for lock installation. The stylist's tools may vary, just make sure you are comfortable with the tools and products based upon this manual's suggestions. In addition, if s/he is a Sisterlock™ Consultant, they better be installing locks with the Sisterlock™ tool! Any other tool, the locks are not considered to be Sisterlocks™, they would be interlocks.

What percentage of your clients are natural? And do you have any pictures of them? What kind of hairstyles or lock installations do you have the most experience with?

Don't let a stylist get away with a general answer. Ask specific questions pertaining to hairstyles or bring pictures and ask her/him how s/he manages the hair through the process. A good stylists will have pictures they proudly want to share with clients and will be able to give details about the products used to get the desired look as well as explain the technique. If there is information shared, contrary to your preference, ask if stylist would be comfortable using your tools, products or equipment. S/he may or may not agree and that's important to note before moving forward. There is nothing wrong with empowering yourself; but, remain respectful.

Can I bring my own products and combs/brushes?

Simply stated, the best tools and products or ingredients are your own tools if they are in line with what has been shared in this manual. Tools should only be used during installation and tightening for lock care.

What products will you use?

The Holistic Hair Care Chapter is the point of reference. Be aware that many commercial product lines used by cosmetologists have unhealthy preservatives. Certified stylists usually implement organic product ingredients. This is a very important question. It is equally important to ask the stylists if you can bring your own products for care and maintenance, if the products used are contrary to the care of your locks. Product disagreement should not negate the technical experience of a stylist who is open to suggestions.

How do you handle client scheduling?

Does the stylist book clients at the same time, rotating while working them into his/her schedule? Or does the stylist focus on one client at a time. Decide what is important to you.

What is your cancellation policy?

Self-explanatory. Make sure the policy fits your schedule in such a way that appointments can be kept in a respectable manner. The stylist's time is very important and so is yours!

How much does it cost? Is a deposit required? How is payment handled? Is there a late fee charged?

Price will vary in different markets. Use the Natural Hair Care Online resource to call around and price for your region[144]. Make sure the payment strategy works for you.

How often do you recommend I come in for salon maintenance?

Remember, locks should only be tightened every 4-6 weeks; but, they can be washed as directed by the stylists or as needed. Frequent washing is fine; however, tightening more frequently than monthly is not. Any stylists that performs tightenings more frequently either does not know or does not have the client's best interest at heart. Simply state that you prefer monthly tightenings only.

How do you think I can improve the health condition of my hair (or maintain it)?

Remember, you may want to wash your hair in between visits. Do you want a stylist that will support your decision, or do you want to be dependent upon the stylist to do everything? It's your choice. Work together for the optimum health of your hair. A stylists that is defensive may not be open to you participating in the care of your hair. Once again, decide what is important to you and make your decision based upon the information that you have gathered.

Remember that attitude is everything. Make the consultation a positive experience by having conversational dialogue that is engaging and non-confrontational. The consultation is a chance to get to know the stylists and vice versa. Be a savvy client, not an irritating one. And, if your involvement in the process seems to be intrusive and to the stylist, the relationship may not work out. The relationship should be complementary and the goal should always be healthy, happy hair.

---

[144]Natural Hair Directory at http://www.thenaturalhaircaredirectory.com/.

From A Stylist's Chair to You

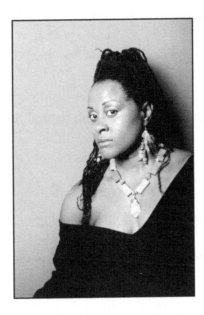

Queen Roshae of Napps Kinks & BBs practices out of Columbus, Ohio
and Phoenix, AZ. She's been practicing since 1989.

It's difficult to get stylists off the stool to give an interview; and, doubly hard to have them open up and share their techniques and business habits. Queen Roshae of Columbus, OH and Phoenix, AZ shares her passion of natural hair which has differentiated her beyond the traditional licensed stylist as a Master Artists. Queen of Napps Kinks & BBs , Queen Roshae shared some of her experience as a licensed professional and care taker of all things nappy.

Why do you exclusively practice natural hair? When did that happen and why did you make that decision?

I have always practiced styling natural hair, but it was not very popular in the Columbus area at the time I entered the professional industry. I exclusively began servicing natural hair after my 3rd child, (2001), after returning home to care for my growing family and began to just do braids and locks at home while on maternity leave. Over a period of time my clientele was also growing and the natural hair demand afforded me the opportunity to continue catering to a growing nappy client.

As a stylist, what tips do you have for customers with natural hair vs loose hair?

The key to nappy hair is MOISTURIZING at every opportunity, and using the proper detangling tools and methods to separate the hair for styling.

What is the biggest mistake you see your customers coming in with?

I often see clients come in with bad information and starting locks every which way: too much product, not the correct size, and no understanding of their OWN hair and journey.

How do you help your customers and continue to have them come to see you?

I begin with consultation first to get a full understanding of the client's wants & needs and visually assess the hair, offering TRUE information on the process, encouragement and information along the way, remaining open for questions and available for follow up services, treating the hair with TLC. Once the trust is established, they stay.

Where did you get trained on the care of natural hair?

My mama, grandmother and trial and error as a big sister, grooming my little sister's hair; and, plenty of practice on my own hair. Then, I just studied what I was doing as an artist and making common sense judgments about what was healthy for the head of hair I was doing. I had the ability to copy styles as a youngster, like an artist, and easily put my own creativity in it.

What was your experience in the cosmetology industry on the instruction of natural hair care?

In 1988-89 there was no curriculum for natural hair care. Further, there was no TRUE study on our hair period, they didn't even teach us how to use pressing combs and marcels when I was in school! I learned a lot by doing and my fellow stylist in the salon, we always shared techniques.

Do you have any additional words of encouragement?

Practice does make Perfect!! *GOD MAKES NO MISTAKES YOU ARE NATURALLY NAPPY.*
-QUEEN ROSHAE

Where can you be found?

NAPS KINX & BB's Urban Day Spa
Queen Roshae, Master Locktician
Business: 614-236-3356
Email:queen@nappskinxbbs.com
http://www.nappskinxbbs.com/

MOBILE UNIT:
Servicing the Phoenix & East Valley Area
614-452-3804

Challenging Barriers
To Economic Opportunity

States with a natural hair styling law, often have the lowest volume of natural stylists. It seems that where legislation abides, an abundance of licensed practitioners do not exist. Within most of these states, the regulations actually exclude stylists from getting a license and practicing legitimately. Or, where the law exists, there's no counter law mandating schools to offer a program in natural hair care, thus shutting natural stylists out. On the contrary, states without registration, or states such as Kansas which only require registration, are more likely to have stylists that are practicing under the auspices of the law, implementing good hygienic practices. Take a look:

As it stands in 2011, there is a natural hair care license in the following states:

Michigan 400 hour Natural Hair Care License, can braid without a license
Illinois 300 hour Natural Hair Care License
North Carolina 300 hour Natural Hair Care License
Washington, DC unspecified number of hours for hair braiding license,1500 cosmetology course
New York 300 hour Hair Braiding license
Tennessee 300 hour Natural Hair Care License, must work under a cosmetologist
Texas 300 hour weaving curriculum that includes hair braiding
Ohio 450 hour Natural Hair Care License
Florida 16 hour health and safety test with limitations for braiders

The following states braiders are exempt from the law:

California
Maryland
Georgia
Wisconsin
Maine
Mississippi
Vermont
Arizona
Connecticut
Kansas
Minnesota
Washington

Presently, the following states require braiders to obtain a regular cosmetology license:

Colorado
Illinois
Iowa
Missouri
Oregon
South Dakota
Wyoming

The states without a specific natural hair law do not differentiate between braiders and natural hair stylists. As a result, anyone that does hair would be expected to obtain a cosmetology license. The bottom line? As those of us that practice the art of natural hair care know, a braider is not necessarily a natural hair stylist. The two may be the same; however, usually they are distinctly different. The archaic laws on the books continually fluctuate and equate a hair braider with a natural hair artist, with both losing their rights. News reports have exposed excessive tension on the scalp resulting in traction alopecia, as well as unsanitary condition, within various hair braiding establishments. This attention often results in law suits and amendments that shut both out of the arena of economic empowerment; impacting natural hair stylists, who usually focus on holistic hair care and locking, not just braiding. In any event, the states where braiders are permitted to work, natural hair stylists often call themselves braiders. In states where there is a natural hair care law, there usually is not a program or a school that offers the program, excluding true natural hair stylists out of their profession. If there is a program, it may be offered in one city within that state, once again, limiting access. The only true, recognizable programs that exist across the union are cosmetology programs which usually require the licensee to obtain a managing license in a program bathed in chemicals with little to no courses covering holistic, natural hair care. Some programs will address limited, braiding techniques. There are progressive states like Maryland that have natural hair schools dedicated to the public and professional with certification options. In addition, other states such as Michigan, Virginia, New York and Georgia have schools with advanced natural hair care offerings with certification options.

If you are truly interested in gaining access to this profession, seeking to legitimize your economic opportunities, it's necessary to lobby a member of congress to draft a bill or an amendment by lobbying and grooming advocates that are passionate about this cause. Once the bill is accepted, the state cosmetology boards are required to carry out the law. It is futile to try to work with the boards who are required to follow the mandate of the law only. Become a natural hair care advocate for justice in your state and petition the legislative branch of government to do something about the pervasive, hypocritical inequities. Licensing is not a bad thing. It's only a bad thing to require people to seek licensing without enforcing schools to provide programs to comply with state legislated mandate. For more information on this important issue please visit and support The Institute of Justice found at http:// instituteforjustice.org. There's much work to do and the fields are ripe for those who care about the cause of empowering those with highly textured hair from the chair to the floors of congress.

INDEXES

Locked vs. Loose Care Overview

Locks	Loose hair
avoid slippery, creamy conditioners	slippery, creamy conditioners are good
split ends encourage tangling and knotting	split ends are not good for hair
coloring can straighten locks, lead to unraveling, bunching	coloring can loosen curl, but fine
less manipulation, the better	less manipulation, the better
constant protective hair style leads to hair growth and retention	hair is exposed to elements, growing hair takes extra protection

Lock Intake Form

A copy should be on file with the locktician, and given to the locker for their file.

Name:

Address:

Phone Number:

Date of Installation:

What name does the new locker prefer?

1. Dreadlocks
2. locks
3. locs
4. Sisterlock's
5. Natti
6. Dreads
7. Other_____

What is the **density of the SCALP**

1. Thick Spacing
2. Medium Spacing(rare)
3. Thinly spaced

What is the **elasticity** of the hair?

If hair snaps and breaks, suggest locker increase water intake 100%. For every pound, they should drink half their body weight in ounces. (100 lb person drinks 50oz/day)

1. snaps and breaks
2. springs back in place

READ

What is the <u>density of the hair?</u>

1   thin
2   medium
3   thick

What is the <u>porosity</u> of the hair?

1   resistant, low porosity(water rolls off the hair)
2   medium(both)
3   highly porous(spongy when wet)

What is the <u>length</u> of the hair?

1   0-2 inches
2   2-4 inches
3   4-10 inches
4   10+ inches

What is the personality of the locker?(chapter 3)
(low maintenance, active, sedentary, type A, relaxed, laid back...)

What is the maintenance personality of the locker?(chapter 3)
(prefers self-maintenance, wants professional assistance, no maintenance and why!)

Are there any professional or religious beliefs that need to be considered?

Financial considerations? Physical challenges?

What is the direction of the lock rotation?

5   Clockwise(towards the right ear)
6   Counterclockwise(towards the left ear)

Product preferences?

Maintenance Preferences?

1. latching
2. palm-rolling
3. latch and roll
4. freeform

Other Notes?

References

Periodicals:

Anderson D, Brinkworth MH, Jenkinson PC, Clode SA, Creasy DM, Gangolli SD. "Effect of ethylene glycol monomethyl ether on spermatogenesis, dominant lethality, and F1 abnormalities in the rat and the mouse after treatment of F0 males." *Teratogenicity, Carcinogenicity, and Mutagenicity.* 1987: 7(2):141-58.

Curtis L. "Toxicity of fragrances." *Environmental Health Perspectives.* 2004 Jun; 112(8):A461.

Darbe PD, Byford JR, Shaw LE, Horton RA, Pope GS, Sauer MJ. "Oestrogenic activity of isobutylparaben in vitro and in vivo.: *Journal of Applied toxicology.* 2002 Jul-Aug;22(4):219-26.

Darbe PD. "*Environmental oestrogens, cosmetics and breast cancer.*" Best Practices and Research: Clinical Endocrinology and Metabolism. 2006 Mar;20(1):121-43.

Exley C, Charles LM, Barr L, Martin C, Polwart A, Darbre PD. "Aluminum in human breast tissue." *Journal of Inorganic Biochemistry.* 2007 sep; 101(9):1344-6.

Kwakman PH, Van den Akker JP, Guclu A, Aslami H, Binnekade JM, de Boer L, Boszhard L, Paulus F, Middlehoek P, te Velde AA, Vandenbroucke-Grauls CM, Schultz MJ, Zaat SA. "Medical-grade honey kills antibiotic-resistant bacteria in vitro and eradicates skin colonization." *Clinical Infection Diseases.* 2008 Jun 1;46(11):1677-82.

McCall EE, Olshan AF, Daniels JL. "Maternal hair dye use and rist of neuroblastoma in offspring." *Cancer Causes and Control.* 2005 Aug; 16(6):743-8.

Neppelberg E, Costea DE, Vintermyr OK, Johannessen AC. "*Dual effects of sodium lauryl sulphate on human oral epithelial structure.*" Experimental Dermatology. 2007 Jul; 16(7):574-9.

Niculescu MD, Wu R, Guo Z, da Costa KA, Zeisel SH. "Diethanolamine alters proliferation and choline metabolism in mouse neural precursor cells." *Toxicological Sciences.* 2007 Apr; 96(2):321-6.

Scaife MC. "An in vitro cytotoxicity test to predict the ocular irritation potential of detergents and detergent products." *Food and Chemical Toxicology.* 1985 Feb; 23(2):253-8.

Stahlhut RW, van Wijngaarden E, Dye TD, Cook S, Swan SH. "Concentrations of urinary phthalate metabolites are associated with increased waist circumference and insulin resistance in adult U.S. males." *Environmental Health Perspectives.* 2007 Jun; 115(6):876-82.

Wojnarowska F, Calnan CD. "Contact and photocontact allergy to must ambrette." *British Journal of Dermatology.* 1986 Jun: 114(6):667-75.

Books:

Cornwell, JoAnne. *That Hair Thing: and the Sisterlocks Approach.* San Diego, Calif.: Sisterlocks Pub., 1997. Print.

Gabriel, Julie. *The Green Beauty Guide: Your Essential Resource to Organic and Natural Skin Care, Hair Care, Makeup, and Fragrances.* Deerfield Beach, FL: Health Communications, 2008. Print.

George, M. Michele. *The Knotty Truth: Managing Tightly Coiled Hair at Home.* 2nd ed. Columbus, Ohio: Manifest Publishing Enterprises, 2007. Print.

R
Rastafarian, 14
right saggital plane, 91
rinses, 24-25
rectangle parts, 75
Robin's Lovin Your Locks, 223
Roll Test, 51
matted roots, 80
root-base, 80
root-bed preparation, 80
rotational planes, 90-92

S
Samson, 14
saponification, 21
scab hair, 47
scalp test, follicle density, 52
seasoned adult stage, 118
settling, 114
shrinkage, 114
single strand twists, 155-167
Sisterlocks™, 205-216
slide test, 50
slipping, 128-129
snipping, 84
specific gravity, 27
splitting, 130
sprouting, 150
square parts,
2-step twist combination method, 90
3-step combination technique, 137
2-strand twists, 65
styles, 240

T
5 in 5 Test, 51
teasing, 47
teenage stage, 115
telogen phase, 45
tensile strength test, 51
tightening method, 78-110
traditional Locks, 208
thymine, 40
triangle parts, 74
Tutankahamen, 14

U
urea preservatives, 20
US Food and Drug Administration (FDA), 18

V
Vanessa's Virtuous Creations, 222

W
Walker, Andre, 43

Photo Credits

About The Author

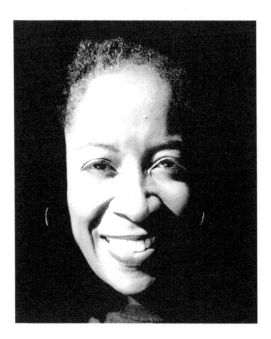

M Michele George resides in Ohio where she is a Biomedical Research Coordinator. With advanced degrees in the biological sciences from Hampton and Clemson University, Michele continues to pursue her passion to free and empower women with the ability to care holistically for their bodies, mind, spirit *and* hair. From her passion, she earned her credentials as a Certified Natural Hair Coach in 2010, in accordance with the United States National Interstate Council of Cosmetology Boards standards for natural hairstyling education to complement her certification in exercise and love of understanding the physiological functions of the hair and body.

Since the release of *The Knotty Truth: Managing Tightly Coiled Hair at Home DIY Survival guide in 2009*, Michele has been busy advocating for natural hair in the Ohio legislature to ensure proper and fair interstate licensing and regulatory laws are congruent for all natural hairstylists, working with international and national natural hair care advisory boards, and traveling to share the mystery of holistic, natural hair care via workshops and seminars for the public and licensed professionals. As an Ohio Board Certified CEU provider, her workshops have allowed licensed stylists to earn professional credits towards their license and the public to gain certification in the area of natural hair care. Michele also consults online, offering her expertise as a Lock Moderator and consult to the Cosmetology Industry.

Michele has made it her quest to empower others by teaching them how to love, learn and care for their own hair. *The Knotty Truth: Creating Beautiful Locks on a Dime! A Comprehensive Guide* is Michele's second book on natural hair care which will enlighten, educate, and inspire all who desire to grow beautiful locks.

Made in the
USA
Monee, IL